MW01095055

5—

15

1/25

Sex When You Don't Feel Like It

Sex When You Don't Feel Like It

*The Truth about Mismatched Libido
and Rediscovering Desire*

Cyndi Darnell

ROWMAN & LITTLEFIELD
Lanham • Boulder • New York • London

Published by Rowman & Littlefield
An imprint of The Rowman & Littlefield Publishing Group, Inc.
4501 Forbes Boulevard, Suite 200, Lanham, Maryland 20706
www.rowman.com

86-90 Paul Street, London EC2A 4NE

British Library Cataloguing in Publication Information Available

Library of Congress Cataloging-in-Publication Data

Names: Darnell, Cyndi, author.
Title: Sex when you don't feel like it : the truth about mismatched libido and
    rediscovering desire / Cyndi Darnell.
Description: Lanham : Rowman & Littlefield, [2022] | Includes bibliographical
    references and index. | Summary: "Distinguishes between love and desire
    to breakdown myths around sex and help readers cultivate an authentic sex
    life"—Provided by publisher.
Identifiers: LCCN 2021048897 (print) | LCCN 2021048898 (ebook) | ISBN
    9781538161708 (cloth) | ISBN 9781538161715 (ebook)
Subjects: LCSH: Sex. | Libido. | Communication in sex. | Communication and
    sex. | Sexual excitement.
Classification: LCC HQ31 .D227 2022 (print) | LCC HQ31 (ebook) | DDC
    613.9/6—dc23/eng/20211012
LC record available at https://lccn.loc.gov/2021048897
LC ebook record available at https://lccn.loc.gov/2021048898

In Memory of
Catherine Carter (1961–2019)
and
Chester Mainard (1953–2007)
Thank You

~

Contents

~

Acknowledgments

Writing a first book is no easy feat, and there were many people behind the scenes that supported me on this journey in a variety of ways.

Let me start with my deepest gratitude to my long-time friend and mentor in sexuality spaces, life, and most recently immigration, Barbara Carrellas. Your encouragement of my work in this space over so many years has meant the world to me and you *continue* to be my greatest ally, collaborator, and writer/righter of life. I love and appreciate you tremendously.

This book wouldn't exist without the initial encouragement of Catherine Deveny, writing coach, dream weaver, and creator of destinies. Thank you for believing in me right from the beginning. Look, I did it!

Thanks to my wife Elle Chase for encouraging me to get this out into the world and to continue despite the odds. Reminding me that writing is hard and editing is even harder, being a voice of reason, empathy, and encouragement.

Thanks to Lorna Hendry for the initial edits and Meg-John Barker for the labor of helping me with flow, context, and placement of content. Your sharp mind and knowledge of the content made traipsing out into my first book feel a lot less daunting. Thanks MJ.

Thanks to Doug Braun-Harvey for listening to my ideas and abstracts and supporting me in clarifying my teachings that form the content of this book. To David Ortmann for the encouragement to write and the support in creating the vision and helping me find my feet in New York City. To Jim Pfaus for the help in understanding the heady brain science. Thanks.

Gratitude to Alex Pitagora, Laura A. Jacobs, Kate Bornstein, and Eric G. Schneider for allowing me to talk about the book at length, its content, its context, and to hear my dilemmas over drinks, dinners, and strolls in the park. Your encouragement and patience are appreciated.

Extended gratitude to Dominic Davies and the gang at Pink Therapy UK for your unwavering support and recognition of my work over the years and faith in this book and its content.

To my mates and colleagues in Australia, the United States, and the UK. You saw and heard me bang on and on *and on* about this book for years. Finally, you get to read it and *maybe* even find it helpful. Hayley Caspers, Emma Eastman, Sam Jacob, Alicia Shevlin, Gala Vanting, Rebecca Wong, Kerrie Thompson-Mohr, Adam Bee, Marc Edwards, Janette Linden, Laurie Liss, Natalie Cohen, Spring Cooper, Christopher Fox, and Belinda Jackson. Thank you for your encouragement and support of my work and transition to the United States.

None of this book would have even been possible without my clients and supporters over the past 25 years. Thank you for sharing yourself with me so deeply that I could turn your wisdom into text to help and support others on their quest for erotic fulfillment.

And to Gomez. My Baby. I love you *so* much. Thanks for reminding me that walking in the park is the best activity ever . . . for bipeds *and* canines.

~

Introduction

> We tend to think of the erotic as an easy, tantalizing sexual arousal. I speak of the erotic as the deepest life force, a force which moves us toward living in a fundamental way.
>
> —Audre Lorde

Feeling lackluster about passion and connection? You're not alone.

We have never been more connected yet less engaged, less satisfied, and lonelier in relationships. In other words: we're fucked; but not how we want to be.

We enjoy personal freedoms our ancestors could have only fantasized about, yet we're lonelier than ever in our intimate relationships. In our hyper-sexed, over-fucked, and under-engaged times, finding purpose and desire in intimacy is tricky. Too often the advice we receive from well-meaning friends, partners, clinicians, and the media remind us that sex is "natural," yet what our relationship with it reflects is to the contrary. Erotic expression is stymied by social and systemic prejudices that inhibit what "natural" flow may be there, and our task of making meaning from the result is far more complex than "horniness" alone. Despite an abundance of sexual information, literally at our fingertips, the gaps between our desires, our values, and how we sustain our connections is corroding our relationships and dissolving our sex lives. When it comes to pleasure, sexual positions and abundant fingering or blow job techniques only take us so far in our quest for erotic fulfilment, because without context and meaning, little else we do matters.

Week in and week out, global publications report the effect bedroom breakdowns are having on our relationships, lives, and even productivity in the workplace. These articles describe how lovers experience loneliness, shame, and pain in their relationships and how frequently these issues show up in the offices of therapists around the world. Marriage is not the bounty of happiness we once believed—if it ever was, and with marriage equality in much of the Western world, LGBTQI+ communities are not exempt. Good Morning America claimed "intimacy anorexia" is a leading cause of sexless marriages, while *Forbes* reminds us that emotional dysfunction at home seriously impacts organizational success.[1] Even the tech industry wants a slice of the relationship pie with couples apps predicted to be the next big thing.[2] The effect of our collective inability to create and sustain nourishing relationships is quite simply, everywhere.

We seek simplicity in a complicated, competitive, and unstable world. Once upon a time, we believed the problem was a lack of access to sexual information. Now, the problem is a lack of knowing *how* to integrate what we find in a never-ending torrent of online possibilities. Spoiled for choice, we have become overwhelmed and untethered from ourselves. Our engagement with dating apps, online porn, and relationships is rarely rooted in connection but, rather, instant gratification. As modern lovers, our challenge is to find value and worthiness in childlike playfulness, but now with the added bonus of adult privilege. In a world where competition and efficiency rules, finding playfulness as erotic purpose is revolutionary.

As far as we know, animals do not place meaning on sex in the way humans do. Animals engage in sexual activity with gay abandon, out in the open with seemingly little regard for who or what is around. While some may have complex mating rituals and some engage in same-sex practices, we're no more certain of their motivations than we were several hundred years ago. Humans, on the other hand, have rather different sex rituals. We have customs, social norms, and cultural and religious expectations. We have meaning at political, social, and individual levels. We have complex familial expectations, relational obligations, and we have very long lives. Most importantly, when allowed, we have eroticism.

Eroticism is the ingredient that distinguishes functional sex from purposeful, connected, meaningful sex in the human domain. Eroticism is sex with the mind switched on. It's where the body, mindfulness, and creativity meet. Without this, sex seems somehow empty and unfulfilling. It's the relationship between our bodies, our practices, and the meanings we place on them that enliven our relationships with Eros to create sex that works and is sustained beyond rudimentary reproduction.

When people seek help with their sex lives in this way, they are often seeking a path through the minefield that is this blend of factors that determine how we register its eroticism. Sex for its own sake is simple enough, but it's when people lose connection and purpose in their sex lives that the cracks start to show and they seek help for something that may have once felt instinctual.

Why This Book and Why Now?
We are *almost* post, post *Men Are from Mars, Women Are from Venus* (an 1980s/1990s best-seller that offered narrow definitions of gender to explain social and relational problems.) Changing the way we talk about sex, gender, pleasure, and power also means changing the way we discuss eroticism, who it's for, and how we access it. Through these pages, I hope to offer you a crucial framework to expand your understanding and discussions of pleasure, power, and gender, while placing it in the context of our modern lives and relationships. You'll be invited to unlearn what you believe about sex and replace it with a useful, more permissive and expansive understanding of your own erotic motivations, to expand your own experiences, relationships, and life.

Rather than just troubleshooting and focusing solely on what's wrong with you, me, or the world, I am especially interested in bringing your attention toward what works—to get you moving, inspired, and engaged. I'll explain the essence of *sexual satisfaction* and not the libido pathology, curable by way of ointments or pills, that we so often see touted in the media or on billboards around town. We'll go deep into sex—emotionally, physically, psychologically, scientifically, culturally, and even spiritually. While I draw on theory and case studies to help you explore further, the true knowledge contained within these pages is not actually within these pages at all. It's inside you. And while feelings are vital and important, they do not tell the whole story. Equally true with science. Number crunching and statistical analysis are useful as signposts but mean nothing when we are in the grip of systemic or personal sexual shame. This book invites you to expand your vision of your own sexuality and, notably, pleasure, to reorient you toward a course of desire and eroticism that brings you meaning, joy, and ease.

Who Is This Book For?

This book is for anyone and everyone interested in sex, desire, and pleasure. It's especially for people who once wanted sex and want to want it again. It's for people who want more sex than their partners and for those who want to understand why they and their partners' desires are different and just never seem to be on the same page. It's for people interested in sex, pleasure, and what makes them tick. It's for people who are interested in really getting more from their sex lives.

Whether you identify as LGBTIQA+, non-binary, poly, kinky, or heterosexual, whether a clinician or layperson, I trust there will be ideas, reflections, and practices in here that will get you thinking, talking, moving, and exploring sex in new and useful ways.

As much as possible, I have tried to include a wide range of genders because, while low libido was once considered simply a "women's problem," over the past ten years I have noticed a huge uptick in men reporting a lack of interest in partnered sex, alongside people whose genders sit outside the current margins. To that end, the implication is the lower desire partner in a relationship is the one who needs to change, so we'll consider how helpful that process is in your particular relationship, while including expanded viewpoints for both higher- and lower-desire partners.

What This Book Is Not

This book is not a sexual trauma recovery manual. I may write one some day, but this is not it. For too many people, struggles with sex *can* stem from trauma and sexual abuse. In the spirit of being trauma-informed, many of the ideas and suggestions we'll explore can be practiced by anyone at any stage in their healing process, but you are invited to be very gentle with yourself should any of these practices trigger you. Go at your own pace and use your discretion.

While the suggestions herein apply to a wide range of people, those who do not or have never experienced any sexual attraction of any kind, to anyone at any time in their lives, and think they may be on the asexuality spectrum may find the content interesting but not especially relevant. This book is also not designed to be a manual for asexuality conversion therapy nor to denounce anyone whose sexuality resides within the asexuality framework. If you are a person who identifies as asexual in a relationship with an allosexual (someone who experiences sexual attraction), you may find some of this content helpful for prompting discussions between you, but you are in no way obliged to act on any of these practices with the expectation of changing your identity or how you feel. This book is also not an homage to so-called sexual dysfunction. It's not an affirmation of medical analyses of sexual performance nor how to make you something you're not. It won't help you enjoy sex that's otherwise unpleasant, boring, painful, or just bad. This book won't help you work out whose fault your sex problems are, but I certainly hope it leaves you feeling more optimistic about them and the wisdom they can uncover when you're willing to work with them.

Finally, this is not a conflict management manual. If you and your partner/s are in high conflict situations frequently, this book won't help you with your attachment issues or chronic arguments. But it might help you see why either of you are struggling with sex and what you can do about it if you want to.

A Note on Language
Throughout this book I use the term "woman" to mean *all* women, "man" to mean *all* men, and "people" to include *everyone*. When I speak specifically of "cis" women or "cis" men, I am referring only to those whose assigned gender at birth matches their identity. When I speak of "non-binary" people, I am referring to people who may identify as neither male nor female or are in some other way gender non-conforming. I use the terms "heterosexual" and "straight" interchangeably to

mean people attracted to an "opposite" sex, though I enthusiastically acknowledge that not all heterosexual people are "straight," as in "conventional"; while many "gay" people can be more "conventional" than they are "queer" or "alternative."

When I speak of "sex" I am referring to *any* activity that arouses, or attempts to arouse, the body and mind simultaneously, with the intention of producing erotic pleasure. It may or may not involve genitals or penetration of any body part with another body part or toy. If I am referring to "intercourse" or "penis-in-vagina" sex, I will refer to it explicitly by name and mean only that.

When I speak of "libido," I am referring to the sensation we usually refer to as "horniness"; in contrast with "desire," which is a significantly more complex state involving mental, emotional, and physical incentives that co-produce imagination and sexual feelings of wanting, longing, and/or passion. The "erotic" and "eroticism" are more ethereal, esoteric, inner-world experiences that complement desire and libido, but also exist in our relationship to life itself. You could say it's the magic ingredient of being alive that gives life its meaning, vigor, and passion.

What's in This Book and How to Use It?
We start by exploring how we came to be in a situation where so many of us are under-fucked and overworked. Or over-fucked and underwhelmed. Then we look at love, romance, pleasure, and desire and take a scuba dive into the leading clinical data on how desire works according to psychologists, sexologists, gender theorists, and neuroscientists.

From there we take a 180-degree pivot and start putting the data to use through a series of practices and reflections designed to help you build and establish *your erotic template*. Your erotic template is essentially the user manual to your unique erotic pleasure. Once you have completed this book you will have the foundations of your personal manual to understand how your desire works, how the desire of your partner/s works, and how you can use and communicate that information to create a fulfilling and joyful sexual life based on what you most value and enjoy. You'll learn:

- about your erotic motivations;
- how to engage your body and quieten your mind during sex;

- how erotic massage works;
- about the value of giving and receiving;
- about taking erotic risks;
- about exploring fantasies; and
- how to talk about what matters with those who matter most.

You'll read examples of how other people just like you navigate issues like these and discover that the problems you face alone are really *not* yours alone, but part of the way our lives are oriented both socially and culturally. As a caveat, the cultural reflections and assumptions contain a strong Western bias, but you can adapt them to suit your cultural context and practice.

You're invited to create a dedicated document that will become the home of your erotic template on your preferred writing device or use an old-school notebook and pen to write your reflections, answer questions, take notes, and otherwise explore the richness of your inner world to make more sense of the outer world. There are many prompts throughout the book including "Time for Reflection" along with other opportunities to consider and reflect. Ideally these practices are to be enjoyed on repeat as you unpack and define your erotic template.

So, as we begin, I'll invite you to initiate your reflections here:

- What if, instead of waiting for desire to take us, we remember how to take it?
- What if the way we want to feel, has been within us all along?

Let me show you how.

CHAPTER 1

~

Everything We've Been Told about Sex Is Lies

Sex is full of lies. The body tries to tell the truth. But, it's usually too battered with rules to be heard, and bound with pretenses so it can hardly move. We cripple ourselves with lies.

—Jim Morrison

Lynn and Rowan walked into my office one evening after a busy work day. Lynn flopped onto the leather sofa and crossed her legs. Her energy was heavy and expectant. As such consultations go, she explained to me that Rowan was a great guy and that their lives and relationship were "pretty good." In fact, she mentioned it several times, as clients often do when they really, *really* want me to know something. Swinging her shoe back and forth from her toe, she breathed a weighty, troubled sigh. And before she uttered another word, tears welled in her eyes. She apologized for this, as for her, the physical response seemed disproportionate to what she was about to tell me. After all, sex isn't a big deal, it certainly doesn't justify tears.

Except for when it does.

When people come to work with me, it's almost always about sex. Or certainly that's where it starts. I've been vocal about the importance of sex for more than fifteen years, so it's no taboo for clients to launch straight into sex discussions with me without the typical posturing that happens between professionals and their clients. And that's how I like it and what has inspired me to write this book. To cut through the sexual malaise, we need to understand not just "what's wrong" but what makes it right—or, at least, better!

Rowan looked down at the floor. Partly ashamed and partly overwhelmed, he seemed familiar with this tableau—and for no reason other than experience, so was I. Here were two lovers, strangers to me, but not to each other, stuck in a bind around sex that is all too common.

"I love him and I love our relationship but I'm just not feeling *it* anymore," she said. "I'm not sure how much longer I can *do* this—*like* this."

"Do what?" I inquired

"Our relationship—the sex I mean. I just don't want it any more. I used to love sex, I used to really look forward to it, but something has died within me. It's breaking Rowan's heart."

"It looks most certainly like it's breaking yours too," I replied. Lynn was visibly distressed by the current situation with her sex life. "What does it say about *you* that you feel like this?" I inquired.

More tears came and she raised her hands to her face to cover the pain she felt. "I feel broken, defective. I shouldn't be feeling like this, but yet—I do."

"*What's* broken"? I whispered to her gently. "*What's* defective?" She looked confused because I didn't immediately concur that *she* was the problem.

All too often, the sex advice we receive from well-meaning friends, lovers, clinicians, and media remind us that sex is "natural," and if we struggle with it, it's because *we* are doing it wrong. By osmosis we believe that sex, and relationships by association, need no attention in order to thrive. That they, unlike everything else in life, exist without us needing to attend to them beyond showing up and hoping for the best. But for anyone who's ever had sex or experienced any kind of complication or contradiction between how they *think* sex should be and how they *experience* it, they know that the alleged simplicity of sex is a lie.

"It's *not* you," I reflected back to Lynn, "because you're actually here and feeling a lot. This doesn't appear to be the temperament of a *bro-ken* woman. So I'm curious; you're *feeling* broken, but yet, *you're* not. Obviously, *something* is broken, and *something* is bothering you, this is true. And you're here doing what anyone would do if they were feeling distressed. That to me looks like someone who's facing something they can't yet make sense of, but not someone who's broken."

She raised her head and looked me right in the eye. "So what *is* this, then?" She asked. "What the fuck is wrong?"

Where the Heck Are We?

Lynn is a modern millennial woman with a typical urban life. Over-worked, moderately paid, and holds reasonably progressive sexual val-ues. She's not ashamed to speak her truth, while her tears reveal both the sadness and frustration she feels—not with Rowan—but with her-self and the situation between them. Rowan is a switched-on guy who cares about how Lynn feels and genuinely aims to please. His enthusi-asm for sex waxes and wanes, but right now he's more concerned about the future of their relationship, with Lynn being so unfulfilled sexually. He can't help but think it's his fault. She can't help but partially agree with him, even though logically, she knows he's done nothing wrong.

Never before has humanity had so much sexual information and access to it at its fingertips. And never before have we been so isolated, conflicted, adrift, and disconnected from our sexuality and pleasure. Despite the slew of titillating and graphic blow-by-blow depictions of sex around us leaving little to the imagination, most of us feel discon-nected from the images we see and the information supplied. Even among those who enjoy sex in their lives, the reflection remains, something's *still not quite right*. It's no longer a case of information being obscured, bodies being misrepresented, or erotic depictions of ourselves not reflected. Instead, there's so much information, yet we do not know what to do with it, nor how to integrate it.

Blaming pop culture for the billions spent on pursuing and prohibit-ing sex is like blaming the apple for being connected to the tree. How is it that sex, the inspiration behind pop culture, fashion, art, music, and porn, manages to be almost invisible in daily conversations when, in fact, everything around us is pointing directly to it?

We are adrift at sea, surrounded by water yet not a drop to drink. Parched and isolated, we crave meaning in pleasure without the wisdom nor skills to make sense of what we see, feel, experience, or crave. The absence of context tricks us into thinking *we* are the defective ones. This book aims to offer meaning, context, and tools to those who struggle to make sense of eroticism and desire in a society awash with facts, stats, and images—on a ship without a rudder.

This information without meaning has no anchor.

After decades of sexual knowledge, diverse representation, and egalitarian pleasure being conspicuously absent from public discussions, the internet has made such information abundant, accessible, and mostly free. For the first time in human history, we are overloaded with knowledge . . . yet we have absolutely no context for it. We are obsessed with sex as a society, but are without tools to make sense of it. We intuitively know that for many of us, eroticism is key to being human, yet everything around it makes *us* feel more defective. After all, sex, like religion, eases the agony of separateness and embodies connection, but we do not treat it with the respect it deserves. It can calm the angst of not being seen. It can validate us and ameliorate feelings of insignificance. It can remind us we are alive and we matter. Sex can also bypass the torture of feeling inadequate. Such majesty has only ever been offered to the masses by religion, until now.

This book is both a call to arms and a systematic breakdown about what lies at the core of human sexuality. In short, this book is about you. Your experience of sex (the physical component), sexuality (its social function in our lives), and eroticism (the pleasures and meaning we make of the acts, thoughts, feelings, and experiences that make us human) and how normal you are in your "abnormal" experience of it. It's an illumination of how your experience of abnormality, discomfort if you will, is actually the grain of sand that creates the pearl we call *desire*.

Everything We Believe about Sex Is Untrue

Sex for procreation, based in love, is a nice idea; and sex in a long-term relationship based on love is an even nicer idea. But the truth is that for most people reading this book, the reasons you have sex are not about making babies and, likely, if you are in a relationship, loving or otherwise, your sex life is anything but nice and simple. Yet this holy grail of "truth" is something most of us hold dear, including well-meaning therapists, despite it not matching our picture of ourselves. Beyond that, the relationship you have with sex is not as straight forward as loving your partner and everything falling into place. Like Lynn and Rowan, if these scenarios were true, few of us would be struggling with sex like we do and none of us would feel so bereft of connection to the very thing society insists is "natural," while simultaneously sanctioning it in ways that make it everything unlike itself.

No other so-called natural act is as heavily policed, legislated against, demonized, scrutinized, or stigmatized as sex. Yet here we all are, swimming around in the soup that insists that *sex is natural.* If we don't buy it, we think there's something wrong with *us,* not the world we live in, our sex education, our ability to explore sex without fear, or our complicated and highly irrational but thoroughly intoxicating relationship with erotic desire.

Desire and libido are synonymous words that describe our relationship with wanting. Usually for sex but, technically, desire can be for anything. Ambition is another kind of desire but far less stigmatized than erotic desire. Ambition for riches beyond the carnal are actively encouraged and rewarded. Money, status, love, success, and education are all markers of a life well-lived. To acquire all of these requires an element of robust desire in action. And desire for multiple and varied life experiences is encouraged as a form of personal development, except when it comes to sex. If we dare show such a relationship with eroticism that centers pleasure over function, we are immediately stopped short. Our entire lives, we are warned against exploring Eros, as if it's very utterance could lead us away from a life of moral or practical fortitude. Yet, once coupled-up, we are duly stigmatized for not having *enough* of it—with no credence nor inquiry into why this might be nor how such a binary of thought may actually be the source of our collective suffering when it comes to the pleasures of the flesh and our relationship to it.

Our sexuality is policed from the day we are born, yet our education to accompany these rules is conspicuously absent. Our gender assigned at birth and our associated orientation may afford us the freedom to know more about it, but none of us are exempt from the scrutinizing gaze that is the erotic shame police and the desire Mafia. There is, apparently, a right way and a wrong way to engage with pleasure, and while no one discusses the nuance nor encourages the skills to tolerate its discomfort, we are all beholden to its rules—that is, until we discover there is another way.

The power and majesty of human sexuality is not respected nor taught with the same reverence we use to teach children about how electricity works. It can be used to power our homes or destroy our lives; it's the user that determines its outcome, but we deliberately omit this knowledge from our most sacred teachings when reckoning with life. It's not until our fingers, moistened with curiosity, are firmly wedged in the socket (pardon the pun) that we realize the power of the force we are plugged into. Without a guide book to make sense of it, we muddle through until the burden has become so destructive that we lose our beloveds, ourselves, and, at worst, our lives. It simply doesn't occur to us we have a choice, because no one has told us we have.

The Fallout

The over-policing of and under-educating about "sex" has created a culture of passivity in our relationship to it. Just like an animal in trauma collapses under overwhelming stress, many of us simply check-out from engaging with sex, leaving its potency and potential unharnessed and unchartered. It's no longer that *we have* sex but, rather, *sex has* us. Without reverence for the magnificence of human sexuality, we find ourselves, like Lynn and Rowan, at war with the erotic. Left unresolved, such internal conflict creates more problems for us than it solves. And when we opt out of developing a relationship with the very thing that brought (most of) us into being, and opportunities to make sense of ourselves in deeply personal ways, such blind spots make for a very messy society and even messier legislation.

Regardless of our sexual identity, erotic discontent manifests as numbness, entitlement, passivity, lack of presence, disconnection, and dissociation, among others. Many of us experience this kind of discord in our relationship with sex and pleasure. Sex is increasingly becoming something "done to us" rather than an expression of creativity, curiosity, or life-force. While perpetually in a dynamic with sex that tells us to "avoid" and "be wary" at worst, or "conquer, empower, and succeed" at best, we have instead become a society in a tug of war with the hopes, struggles, expectations, and anxieties that make us human.

We conceptualize desire as almost exclusively as lust. A physical experience of "horniness" that is held as the marker of ideal sex. A sense of escape from the mundane, as if passively escorted on a magic carpet to a land where pleasure abounds without effort, consequence, or consideration. While horniness is fun and exciting, it's also finite and unreliable. In conceptualizing desire in such a limited way, we remove the more accessible and reliable element of it: incentive.

As long as desire remains a passive experience, we get stuck in a neurotic relationship with its expression. We lose connection with incentive and motivation. The very thing we seek is alive within us as long as we continue to breathe, yet we close-off from it by refusing to accept that desire, like creativity, demands we pay attention long enough to heed its call. While we prioritize everything except the things we *really* want, we remain, like Lynn, in an unfulfilled, neurotic state. Powerless and betrayed by our own lack of inquiry, incentive, and acceptance of what we find there. We wait for desire to take us on a journey, like a bus that never arrives. Disappointed and seemingly stranded, we deduce *we* are the problem rather than the bus. This book invites us, instead, to transform this story by discovering that there is, in fact, more than one way to get to our destination. The bus may be familiar, but familiarity breeds contempt. When eroticism and neurosis become bedfellows, we are called to examine our direction.

The New Paradigm

Throughout these chapters, I invite you to reframe your understanding of sex, pleasure, desire, and all we believe it to be. Whether single or partnered, you'll be lead through a process of sexual discovery that focuses less on "what to think" and "how to be better in bed," and more on working out how and why sex matters to you. Instead of holding *lust* as the sole inspiration for sex, we'll introduce *incentive* as a crucial point of inquiry. We'll seek knowledge from mind and heart but also from the body, in ways few of us as lay people or clinicians value—until now.

Over the many and varied years and continents I have worked with human sexuality, I have uncovered tangible elements and values that sexually satisfied people have in common. This insight forms the understanding of sex I work with today. In working together from this perspective, we prioritize pleasure, we eliminate the need for blame, and get on with the business of change, connection, and growth. We'll take a new path that recognizes individual responsibility and systems of shame, without spending precious energy on solutions that have no problems.

This book is designed to *not* add to the information overload around you. You can find a ton of information on Instagram about giving better blow jobs, how orgasms work, and how to be an expert kisser. There are so many technique-oriented accounts and products out there and yet, still, here we are, uninspired by the sexual status quo.

This book is for the rest of us seeking more than positions and techniques to once again find meaning in sex that has become meaningless.

It's designed to teach you *how* to make sense of the information, and yourself, in a world that is full of "panicdotes" and clickbait headlines about sex that take you further from where you want to be. Instead of telling you what's wrong, with your permission, I'll attempt to teach you how to grow into your edges, how to trust yourself more, how to make sex easier, how to accept what you cannot change, and how to make sense of humanity's obsession with sex that shows little interest in making a connection to it.

Even for Me . . .

I came to this work in human sexuality through recognizing the value of playfulness and risk. I recall, as a child, observing how miserable so many adults were. Of course, I had no evidence of their misery, but I felt it in my bones that, somehow, they had lost touch with the joy that comes to us more naturally as children. These adults in the gray suits and soured hearts traded playtime for tight collars and pleasure for obligation without even realizing they had a choice. Previous generations pursued lives devoid of self-inquiry, in favor of "doing the right thing." I vowed to myself I would never let this happen to me, and although I too live with pressure, recovered trauma, anxiety, and sadness from time to time, it is not the totality of my story as an adult seeking pleasure. I am perpetually interested in how pleasure remains buoyant, in sex and in life, even if it seems out of reach to me in any given moment. Like Lynn, the feeling of being defective is a powerful distraction from learning new truths about sex and pleasure; yet, there is something about the spaces between the points of joy and anxiety that keep eroticism fresh. I am especially keen to explore and observe how pleasure and other personal values form an incentive when our wishes, difficulties, shortcomings, and expectations derail us. I am interested in teasing out what keeps us from feeling playful, curious, abundant, and satisfied, and reframing what we find there.

In the next chapter we'll consider the role of pleasure and how it informs how we teach, learn, and experience sex. We'll look at who gets access to it and what the effect of that is on our personal lives and in our bedrooms. Be sure to get your chosen notebook ready, if you haven't already. Pour yourself a drink and settle in. I'll see you there.

CHAPTER 2

~

Why Pleasure Matters

Let go of who you think you're supposed to be.
Embrace who you are.

—Brené Brown

In this chapter we'll begin by considering one of the most important elements of desire, often overlooked by medicine, the media, and our daily conversations: pleasure. For some reason or other, pleasure is not a default but an afterthought when we talk about sex, while function, performance, and frequency overwhelmingly tend to be front and center. The emphasis here is on measuring up, sizing down, stepping up, being hot, getting wet, acting sexy, being attractive, and, certainly, sexual *enough* . . . but not too much (though no one can really tell us how much is or is not quite *enough*). And of course, most of these ideas are introduced to us from a very young age through our experience of our gender and the sexual freedoms that come with that. These ideas are so embedded that we've been tricked into thinking they're *natural* . . . but nothing could be further from the truth.

Like it or not, sex is all around us. From social media accounts, lingerie ads, beer ads, and sports matches to religious ideologies, places of worship, personal development communities, fashion marketing, pop music, and porn. Even conversations with friends, co-workers, or people on the street can easily divert to sex (though not erotic), conversations like political scandals with interns and such, the implications of "pussy-grabbing," navigating dating apps, and even whether or not the #metoo movement has "gone too far" (as I have been subjected to on at least several occasions). It's likely that you or someone in your circle has talked to you about their or their partner's cheating, or you flipped thorough a magazine at the doctor's office that showcased an article about sex positions, squirting, dating techniques, or the best-ever blow jobs. Maybe your pastor, rabbi, guru, lama, or imam has given you strict codes of conduct about sex, your gender, or the role of both in marriage—after all, this trifecta informs so much of how people experience sex, their bodies, and their desires. You've likely been inundated with information about drugs to make you or your partner last longer and perform better, or surgeries to boost and lift, or ointments that reduce pain to go harder, faster, deeper and longer—usually for the benefit of *one* of you, rarely for both—and while pleasure is implied, it's not guaranteed. Dating tropes in movies and TV shows usually follow the same format of the bumbling idiot (usually a man) on a quest and the cool, reserved, graceful "prize" whose pleasure is to "be desired." Or the distancer / pursuer combo, where the distancer (usually a woman) earns her status by disengaging from her pleasure, acquiescing to his and letting herself "be caught," but only once the pursuer has proved his worth. Sometimes this ends in marriage—allegedly the most ideal outcome—but sometimes, especially if the distancer gives in too soon ("slut"), or the pursuer is too horny ("sex addict"), they'll get their comeuppance, which is often grizzly and shameful, because they colored outside the lines and "deserved" it. And in mainstream porn, the most stigmatized of media for its explicit portrayal of pleasure, women are *always* there to please men, ironically, whether men are in the scene or not. And men, gay or straight, only have *one* way of being pleased: orgasm. While porn gets the worst rap for its tedious gender portrayals, from these examples we can see that the apple in this case hasn't fallen far from the tree. Our tropes about sex, pleasure, gender, and power are everywhere and they're all strikingly similar whether in scripture, on the street, or in porn. From the Vatican to Vegas, from Hollywood to Disney, we desperately want sex and relationships to be easy. No nuance. No complexity. No problems. It's natural. Sound familiar?

These cultural stories tell us over and over how sex should be, how much is too much or not enough, when it should happen, how it should happen and what happens if you step out of line. This torrent of daily messaging about sex informs so much of what people struggle with in their sex lives without them even realizing it. Across communities, cities, and cultures, there is little variation on these ideas. Some may be slightly more liberal than others, but ultimately all kowtow to a central notion of "real sex" as intercourse and pleasure as implicit—never explored or unpacked and embedded within that singular act. Because most of us *only* learn sex through these narratives—without any other reflective or reflexive frameworks—it never occurs to us to question them. We are told on repeat that sex is natural and therefore there is no need to learn, explore, or query it. And beyond that, the implication is that the pleasure that comes from sex is universal. In other words, if one person likes a thing, in this way, at this time . . . surely, then, the other people they want to do it with like that thing too, right?

Not really.

As we move along in this work you will be invited to reflect on an abundance of physical activities that may inspire desire, but also activities that actually invite and center *pleasure*, the cousin of desire that is often implied but misunderstood. Pleasure-based activities may or may not be explicitly sexual and may or may not involve genitals, penetration, nudity, and so on. That is to say, *pleasure* comes from many activities and aspects of life that can inspire desire and eroticism. But many of these may not fit into categories we traditionally associate with "real sex" (a.k.a. intercourse), or are considered simply precursors to "real sex," despite many people finding them *more* fulfilling and satisfying than any "real sex" act itself.

The trouble with dismissing the value of *pleasure* over the notion of "real sex" is far reaching and powerful. Such legislation, whether social or actual, corrals us into believing there is sex that is *good* and *right*, and sex that is *bad* and *wrong*. It allows us to justify and privilege certain kinds of sex, or certain kinds of relationships or sexual contexts, while dismissing or criminalizing others based on an "objective" moral hierarchy. It coerces and pressures people into doing things they may

Time For Reflection: What Is Pleasure?

Pleasure is a complicated word. For some of us, it rolls off the tongue. For others, it's riddled with sleazy connotation of indulgence and superficiality. Before we dive into pleasure and its relationship to sex, let's get to know pleasure—non-sexual, non-explicit—on its own. Open a page in your notebook and begin by considering these questions:

1. How would you describe your relationship with pleasure?
2. Is pleasure important to you? Does it seem frivolous or a waste of time?
3. Was pleasure considered valuable when you were growing up?
4. What did you do today that was pleasurable?
5. What did you do this week that was pleasurable?
6. Who else did it involve?
7. What circumstances made it pleasurable? (e.g., time, money, sensations, words, feelings, movements, gestures, etc.)
8. Who helps you create pleasure in your life?
9. How do they do it? (e.g., they allow me to have free time; they listen to me; they don't pressure me; they compromise; they give me money; they offer my favorite sex acts to me; etc.)
10. Because of this pleasure in my life, my life is more . . .
11. Without this pleasure, my life would be less . . .

Go easy on yourself as you open the Pandora's box that is pleasure. For some of us, taking the time to offer ourselves pleasure is challenging. For others, it's a right-of-passage. No matter where you are in your relationship with pleasure, allow yourself to consider the degree to which you welcome and make space for it in your life. As we work though this book, you will be invited to reflect on pleasure in many ways. You can come back to these questions anytime, over and over again.

not like, want, or enjoy because the need to fulfill a social script about "real sex," and thus be perceived or indeed perceive themselves as "normal," often feels more powerful than the self-inquiry of subjective, moment-by-moment pleasure.

Case Study: Clinton
Clinton was a young man in his early thirties who came to see me after a breakup from a passionate relationship. He still missed and pined for his previous lover, but also recognized the relationship was complicated, erratic, and wearing down his mental health. Eventually, the relationship ended and Clinton was devastated.

In the pursuit of moving on, Clinton, like many others, turned to Tinder. As someone identifying as bisexual and keen to also explore gender and kink, Clinton found the dating app a ready and easy source of contact. Despite being a conventionally good-looking man, there was something cautious about Clinton that made him approach dating more mindfully than most men his age. The challenges of modern-day masculinity and the performance of "being a man" took their toll on Clinton, and as much as he felt "OK" with his gender, he was not OK with being perceived as a predator by women, or having to do the chase or perform his desire or dominance when dating men, or anyone else for that matter. He found navigating the space between introduction and hookup *especially* challenging. So many social scripts. So many expectations. So much anxiety and so little room to relax. Clinton often lamented that hookups and casual sex would leave him feeling "shredded." The pressure of having to flirt, to impress, and to strut like a peacock did nothing to enhance his enthusiasm for sex; if anything, it greatly reduced it.

"Sex, for me, is always much better in a relationship," he explained. "I feel like I can be myself, let my guard down a bit, and really let myself go. The way it is now, when I'm single, I feel vigilant. I'm always performing and checking myself. I can't relax and then I lose my erection. There's no pleasure in that for me and I leave the situation feeling torn apart."

Despite Clinton's frustrations with the status quo of gender, sexual expectations, and hookups, it became increasingly apparent that, for Clinton, intimacy was a core condition he needed in order to be able to let go and enjoy sex. Sure, he could function without it. A bit of

Viagra and a few beers for courage would sometimes get him over the line. But this was the exact ritual he hated, having to puff himself up to get himself off. Masturbation was a more appealing alternative. But the difference here was that Clinton didn't want to simply "get off." He wanted to connect, not necessarily in a long-term relationship, but he needed a level of intimacy, even in a hookup, that would allow him to be able to focus his attention on pleasure rather than what he was doing, how long he would last, or what his partner was thinking of him.

The struggle between wishing he were more "casual" about sex, like many of his friends, and paying attention to what his body and intuition was telling him was challenging. He was caught between wanting to be free and wanting to be free-of-it. His mind was telling him he needed to get over it while his body was telling him exactly what it craved and needed in order to be satisfied. With this knowledge firmly in his grasp, the quandary for Clinton immediately changed from, *How can I be more comfortable with hookup sex?* to, *How can I be more comfortable with myself?* At once, he realized the satisfaction he was seeking wouldn't come from finding the perfect partner but by being the person he needed to be for himself—before, during, and after sex.

Clinton realized that when we focus on distinguishing *pleasurable* from *less pleasurable* sex, rather than how to do it *right*, the emphasis is much more on our relationship to ourselves, how we connect to our truths, our pleasures, and our expression, than giving an Oscar-winning performance. This includes our feelings about ourselves, what we are doing and how, the connection between us, the moment and so much less about bending to convention. In other words, *it ain't what you do, it's the way that you do it* that brings the pleasure we want from sex. When we are able to orient ourselves away from the pressures of sex solely as a performance, like "real sex" tends to be gauged, we open ourselves up to being able to center and privilege *pleasure* as a motivator for not only sex, but also for joy, connection, and so many of the other things many of us hope to gain through sex and sex alone.

Clinton's experience is common for many men, especially men who struggle with sex and long for something more. But do not be fooled that his is a gender problem. This is a contextual problem that affects all of us based on the stories we believe about sex, how we experience ourselves, our bodies, our genders, and so on. Later in this chapter we'll look more at what research thinks about pleasure, desire, and gender, but for now let's examine, like Clinton, how pleasure works for us.

In chapter 7 we'll explore a lot more of what makes sex pleasurable, memorable, and even amazing according to research and practice. But for now, our focus is on distinguishing pleasure for its own sake, including how pleasure is or isn't afforded to us, as determined by social scripts around sex and gender. And on understanding its impact on how our bodies interact with our thoughts, feelings, and other bodies to perform sex *right*, despite how pleasure operates within us as individuals. In the same way it's understood that "real sex" means penis-in-vagina intercourse, it's also equally assumed that the point of sex, any sex, is to have an orgasm. This means that we can end up getting hyper-focused on the quality of sex, which is measured by the occurance and quality of an orgasm. And to that end we can also sidetrack our own pleasure by making sure we "achieve" an orgasm or making sure our partner has at least one, if not multiples, as a way to boost our ego, but not necessarily their pleasure. To be clear, I am not anti-orgasm, heck I have online courses about the subject because they do matter and they are pleasurable. And traditionally, orgasm has been very much in the realm of men, so for anyone else of any other gender to claim space at the orgasm table is both political and personal, if it's about *your* pleasure. Nevertheless, even when modern sex-positive culture creates pressure to have them, no one can really say, with any degree of ease or authority, *why* they really matter so much or *what* they even mean. The thing is, pleasure comes in many forms, and our motivations for sex—our desire for it—has a lot more to do with the idiosyncratic process of our capacity for pleasure than it has anything to do with a culturally sanctioned orgasm, no matter how "explosive" or "empowering" it may feel. At the end of the day, when we are trying to find our way back to sex, back to desire and enthusiasm, as sexologist Emily Nagoski says, "pleasure is the measure."[1]

Pleasure, Diversity, and Desire: Who Gets to Desire or Be Desired?
Knowing what brings you pleasure or fulfilment makes it easier to get. Spending time considering what situations and contexts bring you the most pleasure is a very helpful key in understanding your own individual patterns of pleasure and desire. Cis women, by and large, are most often at the mercy of lower libidos, or certainly more context

Time for Reflection

Open your notebook to a new page, get a pen and a drink, and relax a while.

Allow yourself to recall a time you engaged in some kind of erotic or sexual activity that was especially enjoyable one time, but less so on another. As a note, do not choose something that is too traumatic or upsetting to think about. An example could be a kiss that was incredible one time, and a kiss (with the same or different person) that you wanted to escape from. Or, perhaps some kind of hand sex that was amazing one time and pretty mediocre another. Whether a partnered or solo activity, allow yourself to recall that *same* activity, but in these two very different contexts. As you recall both experiences try to recall as much detail as possible and capture as much as you can by writing. It needn't be an essay; bullet points are fine. Try dividing the page into two columns to compare and contrast the two experiences, writing about one aspect that was great in one column and the same aspect that was not in the other. If writing is not your thing, try drawing it.

Consider things like: What was the location? What was happening before? How did it start? How were you feeling emotionally and physically? What was on your mind? How did things proceed? What were your responses as things proceeded? How did it end? How did you feel after? Compare the differences in experience and notice what stands out about the two situations and why one was more pleasurable than the other even though it was the exact same activity? On the enjoyable side, many people notice things like Clinton did; their headspace at the time, how comfortable they felt with the person or the activity, how confident they were feeling about their body, how present and in tune with their body they were. But on the less enjoyable side were things like worrying about measuring up in terms of size, lasting long enough, wetness, hotness, and so on. Or when the activity was goal-oriented and performance-based, what made it less enjoyable was worrying about their skill level, whether the other person knew they didn't know what they were doing, the degree to which they acquiesced or felt pressured. By discovering what brings you more pleasure, you're well on your way to understanding more about desire.

driven or responsive libidos than men, according to research (more on that in chapter 4). But let's remember also that it was assumed, until fairly recently, that cis women didn't really even *like* or *want* sex; and if they did, the imperative was for reproduction and not pleasure. This matters a lot because the way we are taught—in our education and social messages—to respond to sex, pleasure, and our bodies, is, as we considered earlier, very gendered. For example, straight cis men *never* hear that their bodies are:

- disgusting;
- smelly;
- the cause of someone's violence or lack of self-control;
- injured or killed for wearing the wrong thing or being in public after dark; or
- enjoying particular sex practices, solely "because they were abused as children."

Similarly, heterosexual cis women never hear that they should be:

- out "sowing their wild oats";
- seeking to punch above their weight;
- affirmed for being single and successful at thirty-five, forty, or fifty; or
- getting congratulated for "doing" the entire team!

In the 2020s, cis women may be *doing* these things, but most still tend to keep it quiet, especially if they are parents, lest their reputations become untethered. Nowadays, cis women are allowed to want sex rather than solely be wanted *for* sex, but usually only in an ongoing relationship (and usually only after she has known her prospective partner for a little while). The threat of "asking-for-it" is only a breath away should she dare express her desire or enjoyment of her own body. The default still implies that her sexuality is there for others and neither for herself nor her pleasure alone. Imagine the effect this has on her capacity to enjoy sex! Cis men are expected to *want* sex and get horny at the drop-of-a-hat. They're told through narrative and action that sex is *for* them, for the taking. While many recognize this is not true, the power of cultural inheritance is such that this remains a privilege all women have yet to access. It's not a free-for-all though. Too much sexual energy and too many partners, and men run the risk of being called a "sex addict"—the pathologized "boy" equivalent of a slut or a whore. And while there may be some basis for gendered sexual stereotypes, to reduce something as nuanced as pleasure and desire down to only two options determined by gender is a gross oversimplification.

The jury is still out on what makes men and women different (or the same) in many of our behaviors, and sex is no different. Each year, new ideas are put forward about what gender is, who benefits from it and how it plays out among different racial groups, cultures, and socioeconomic groups. Modern gender theorists suggest that "male" and "female" are only two of a whole variety of genders any of us may embody at any one time[2] and that gender is determined by so much more than our hormones or our genitals. But when it comes to sex, pleasure, and desire, the gendered assumptions remain pretty static. "Men are like this—women are like that," and so on. Somehow, we have become pretty invested in men and women being not only different but *opposites*, because it helps us make sense of ourselves and our complicated (heteronormative) world. Let's look at some examples here of how this plays out in our daily conversations about gender.

Men	Women
spontaneous	responsive
testosterone	estrogen
hot	cool
chasing	chased
fire	water
yang	yin
giver	taker
doer	done
initiator	recipient
active	passive
desiring	desirable
pleasure-oriented	connection-oriented
lust	love
primeval	ethereal
embodied	otherworldly

The implied solution is—if only one were more like the other, all our problems would be solved. But of course, it's not that easy. Those of us in same-sex relationships experience the same dilemmas and differences in libido, because *desire* is a human quandary, a relational quandary, and a contextual quandary *including* a gender quandary. A large body of evidence suggests that cis men experience physical sexual desire more strongly and more frequently than cis women; however, it is not clear whether sexual desire is *truly* gendered or if gender differences are influenced by how sexual desire is activated and assessed.[3] In other words, we don't know if so-called sex drive (more on this in chapter 5) is *really* stronger in cis men, or, if they were *not* the "standard" against which "normality" is measured, how different the results would be. As long as we default to cis men's sexuality being the norm and cis women's sexuality as "men's sexuality—lite," we may never get an accurate assessment.

The cat and mouse game of sex, sometimes referred to as "polarity," is part of the thrill of connection in sexual partnerships, which over time can become a source of conflict in relationships. Many ancient Eastern perspectives on sex suggest that these "masculine" and "feminine" qualities are present within all of us but have little to no bearing on our biological sex or gender assigned at birth. In other words, we can and do all embody these qualities in different situations and different times in our lives. Just like Clinton from earlier in this chapter and his longing for connection, he was wedged into a role he simply hadn't auditioned for. It's this assumed polarity, a forced binary that is often suggested as the source of both resistance and attraction in eroticism, regardless of the genders of the partners. While these interpersonal qualities are often gendered in our social attitudes, these things are also *universally* a source of conflict in sexual relationships regardless of gender. Who initiates what we do and who is desirable are *relational* problems, not a gender problem. But in trying to make sense of ourselves, we apply gender to qualities that are in fact quite human. When we *genderize* the sexual experiences in our lives, when we take privileges over others because of a social belief, we prevent ourselves from being able to make room for the robustness that is our sexual expression.

The truth is pleasure and desire are so much more nuanced and complex than modern interpretations of gender can consider, and even though gender roles and stereotypes have been and continue to be blasted time and time again, when it comes to sex and desire, old habits, values, and beliefs die hard.

The Science Behind Gendered Desire

Cis Men

Very little study is done on what *actually* turns cis men on, how they experience pleasure, and what motivates them to have sex despite the increase in cis men seeking psychosexual therapy for their waning or non-existent libidos. In terms of desire, research disproportionately reduces cis men's sexuality to testosterone and erections—decreasing their role in sex to little more than coin-operated sex machines. The default assumes they are hardwired for sex at all times. That they are the initiators of sex with no need to be *the desired*. That *to desire* is a masculine "trait" and inherited solely by its fusion with masculine identity. Any man, of any orientation, not displaying it is called to question not only his sexuality but also his masculinity; as if there's only *one way* to express eroticism when you have a penis or a masculinized body. Because sex, erections, libido, and power are inextricably linked with masculinity, to be soft is to be "unmasculine" and associated with being weakened or having lesser status. It doesn't make him a woman, it simply makes him "unmasculine"; a reject that has no home in a culture that only tolerates two opposing genders. To want to penetrate, or "top," is masculine, to want to be penetrated, or "bottom," is feminine, with little space between these poles to explore pleasure for its own sake. In opening oneself up to self-inquiry like Clinton, one must initially confront the fear of self-emasculation, implying a loss of status, a form of social rejection, and a source of shame. In queer men's communities, where explorations of multiple masculinities are at their most robust, the visibility of men calling for "masc" (short for masculine) in their dating profiles reinforces the idea that being anything other than "masc," even outside the heterosexual world, is simply not OK.

When men's expression of sexual pleasure is derailed in these ways, there is less incentive for them to explore what *really* turns them on, brings them joy, or enables them to find erotic fulfilment. Evidence suggests that the majority of cis men's libidos are affected by:

- feeling desired;
- exciting and unexpected sexual encounters;
- intimate communication;
- rejection;
- physical ailments and negative health characteristics; and
- lack of emotional connection with partner.[4]

But when trait-based expectations of sex and libido remain unquestioned in intimate relationships, they can lead to cis men feeling lonely in their sexual and gender expression, contributing to further withdrawal from engaging in sexual activities. The effect of such narrow understandings of pleasure, desire, and gender has disastrous effects on intimacy and connection, particularly within relationships where acting "masculine" is an obligation.

Beyond this, evidence confirms that cis men in long-term relationships also experience a more fickle relationship with desire. Where raging lust may have once lived, a tamed beast may be more susceptible to emotional and contextual interference, and to experiencing more inconsistencies in his sexual interests.[5] In other words, if ravenous desire once *seemed* the norm, it's very easily transformed into something more contextual and sensitive in a long-term relationship. When a man experiences his sexuality only through a gendered lens of lust and initiation, committing to a relationship could be interpreted as a threat to his masculinity. Perhaps this is the reason cis men are so often accused of "commitment-phobia" and other such juvenile ideals of human sexuality. Not because they are afraid of commitment, but rather the loss of status they may experience due to their fragile erotic identities.

From a clinical perspective, the bias in cis men's sexuality research assumes that lust is a given with little enquiry into its origins. The story is men are simple. Research is funneled into performance-enhancing drugs, like Viagra and Cialis (which promote erection but not desire), instead of pleasure, desire, and motivation. The lack of discussion regarding "what men want," tricks us into thinking the riddle has already been solved. It mustn't be important because no one is talking about it. It is assumed that *all* men (queer and straight) want sex and the problem exists only when they can't because their erections are unreliable. It also assumes that for men to enjoy sex they must be hard, they must be able to "perform," and, if they get that right, they are *real* men and sexually satisfied.

Cis Women
Research into cis women's sexuality is effectively, and predictably, the opposite. The focus is on problems and disorders of desire and arousal and very little on their authentic pleasures and satisfaction. What it shares in common with men's research is the focus on *performance* (doing it right) rather than feeling and motivation. It is assumed that the traits we associate with cis men and sex are desirable for cis women too. Feeling horny, liberated, and confident are likable qualities, but only to a point, remember? A woman who's too sexually awakened is . . . asking for it. But while so-called sex-drive is the norm, clinical studies will continue to focus on interventions designed to make cis women "better," more liberated and free—that is, more like men.

The vast majority of studies that explore "what women want" show diverse results. This unfortunately compounds the narrative that women are complex. But, as we have seen, it's not women who are the problem but rather the normalized concepts of sex, pleasure, and gender that don't include them. It could be argued that desire problems are not gendered at all, but rather the result of the way we conceptualize libido at the outset.[6] In other words, the differences and similarities among genders in regard to our sexuality are a thing. The trouble is, they are not celebrated and barely understood.

As described, we're more interested in how sex *looks* rather than how it feels. We want to make sure we're *normal*, doing it right—with little trust in our own instincts about what feels good (there's a pile of reasons for that, but we'll get to that later). It's no surprise that our clinical investigations produce inconclusive results, because incentives and triggers are reduced to gender traits while our sexual motivations aren't valued or, worse still, erased because there's no context for a new kind of normal.[7]

Non-Binary and Trans Folx and Pleasure and Desire

Unsurprisingly, little research has been done on the sex lives of trans and non-binary people, and, as a result, little is known outside of these communities about not only their sex lives but also their pleasures, interests, and desires. Where correlates of sex hormones such as testosterone have impacted a spike in libido in all genders, it's inconclusive as to how much it's due to introduced hormones (if there are any) and, specifically for trans folx, how much is due to transitioning and feeling better about oneself in general. That said, desire in trans women was shown to decrease in the majority after the intervention of hormones and / or surgery, but it increased in the majority of trans men. This is not conclusively true, however, as the studies were limited in their capacity to gauge the individual's relationship to desire prior to transitioning. Such results yield subjective interpretations. Interestingly of the trans women interviewed, few found the decrease in desire a hindrance or a disappointment[8] largely due to overall life satisfaction increasing as a result of living a more fulfilled life. This was echoed by psychotherapist and sex therapist Lucie Fielding's findings in her book *Trans Sex*,[9] where she notes how the defaults of cis normativity have a devastating effect on the pleasure capacities of people whose bodies exist outside the gender mainstream. While most sex research and sex advice tends to center around the experiences of cis people (both straight and gay), those whose bodies deviate from the norm, whether through gender, disability, or size, are still forced to do the extra work of extrapolating what pleasure looks like for them, without sex being reduced to something as basic as hormones and injections alone. Fielding goes on to consider that when indeed the effects of hormones, for those taking them, create changes to their bodies and their horniness levels, people may experience both bliss *and* devastation simultaneously, as the trade-off of having to lose or gain sexual desire as a price to pay for their gender euphoria. She explains that sometimes this shift may be less of a trade-off and perhaps more of a shift in their erotic template; something that happens to all of us through our lives, yet something that's remarkably still overlooked by sex research and sexual medicine.

As we reach the end of this chapter, go easy on yourself as you begin to think about dissecting pleasure, desire, power, and gender. This isn't about replacing one set of rules about sex with another, only to keep you trapped even further. Instead, we'll begin to build our own erotic templates and learn how they evolve and shift as we learn more about ourselves, what we like, what matters, and how to best share that with those who need to know. When rebuilding our sexuality from the ground up, we are unpacking thousands of years of conditioning. "But it's worth it 'Because you're worth it,'" as the saying goes. The next chapter will take you further into this investigation as we take a closer look at desire and how it's informed by pleasure and so much more. See you there.

CHAPTER 3

~

What Is Desire?

Desire is a teacher: when we immerse ourselves in it without guilt, shame, or clinging, it can show us something special about our own minds that allows us to embrace life fully.

—Mark Epstein, *Open to Desire*

In the last chapter we unpacked pleasure, who gets to have it and how gender plays a role in how we talk about sex, while consistently avoiding talking specifically about pleasure. In this chapter, we'll explore what desire means—socially, personally, and even politically—and, more importantly, why it matters, especially if it's something we struggle with. We'll unlearn how desire is spoon-fed to us broadly and also journey into our own deeper individual understandings of desire. Together we'll consider how accurate and helpful these ideas and beliefs have been, and continue to be, for us as we start to explore the impact of our desire education and its effect on our sex lives and relationships.

34

Conceptualizing Desire

- If you could take a pill to make yourself eat a vegetable you don't particularly like, would you?
- If you could take a pill to make yourself watch sports when you were actually more into painting, would you?
- If you could take a pill to make grocery shopping more exciting, would you?

If you don't particularly like something or you don't want to do it, in most circumstances we would agree that this is perfectly reasonable.

Except when it comes to sex.

We live in a society that tells us that if we don't want sex there is something wrong with us. We are broken or damaged in some way. We become afraid that it may spell disaster for our relationships or will change the way our lovers or potential lovers may feel about us.

Desire for sex is an expected yet highly inconsistent element of modern relationships. So many clients have come to me to discuss their relationship with desire over the years, I could almost have started a practice based solely on the exploration of desire.

When we reflect on desire, many of us arrive at synonyms like joy, abandon, and aliveness. But for others still it can also indicate obligation, belonging, and feeling "normal." Sexual desire is synonymous with freedom, passion, and youthfulness. It's a concept that we connect to culturally because we are *expected* to feel it, frequently, consistently, reliably, especially if we are in an intimate relationship. It is, we are told, a marker that shows us we are with the right person. That they bring this out in us. It's passive. Something that happens *to* us rather than something we build or create together.

But for many people, desire is experienced as anything but youthful abandon. For many it shows up as pressure or shame. Somehow the great expectations we have of desire and sex in intimate relationships do not manifest in our bodies the way we would like or expect them to, especially if we have been together a while. Clearly there is a gap between the ideal we've been offered and the reality many of us experience. And that magical place between those two points is unique to each of us, depending upon our mental, emotional, and physical resources.

Desire is so much more than simply yearning for sex. Desire speaks to our connection with Eros, the mysteries of the flesh, the possibility of fulfilment, and what sex means to us. It speaks to a connection to our partners but, more importantly, a connection to ourselves. And it also speaks to freedom. A sense of weightlessness that transcends the every day. An ability to give ourselves over to something that extends beyond logic and invites us to surpass the mundane, the practical, and the stable, and to engage with life from a place that is less rational and more visceral.

Scientists and mystics have tried to measure, quantify, and calculate how desire works for many years. They have come up with theories but no definitive answers. This suggests there is no proven method for cultivating and maintaining desire. It remains evasive, illusionary, and consistently unreliable. Yet, especially in Western cultures, we elevate desire to almost a divine, magical status. It *is* magical and it *does* represent so much that is good in life—for many, but not all of us. We cannot agree on what it is, how it feels, how it works, or what it does, but it is often present in discussions of sex and pleasure, both in and out of sexual relationships.

For this reason, the definition of desire in this book will be constructed by you. Your reflections will establish how desire sits and feels, why it matters to you, and its purpose in your life.

Know Thy Desire

Desire is many things to many people. When asked to describe desire, our vocabulary is rich and diverse. It needs to be. Because when we are able to know desire for ourselves, we are better able to accept it within ourselves. We are better able to understand:

- its ways;
- how it operates;
- what makes it more or less present; and
- how to communicate it to those who need to know more about us and our relationship with it.

When I ask people to describe desire, some common themes emerge:

Freedom
- creative chaos
- love without logic
- risky adventures
- fun, excitement
- exploration
- playfulness

Visceral
- needing, can't get enough of . . .
- wanting sex with someone, what turns you on
- passion, lust, sexiness
- electricity
- really wanting something, sexual desire, lust, longing
- unbridled passion
- feeling horny when I was younger
- wanting
- richness, physicalized emotion
- soft, wet, hot
- passion, urge, excitement, exploration, fun
- physical attraction
- foods, sexual turn-ons

Connected
- warm intimate contact, connection
- warm feelings, wish for intimacy
- feeling sexually aroused and also interest (emotional, mental, and physical) in being intimate with partner
- being in tune with needs, being present, fully experiencing the fun of sex
- wanting to be sexual with another person, in whatever form sex takes

It's interesting to note that few people connected desire to anything easy or simple. The descriptions involve an element of either abandon or connection. Nor did they use words like "nice," "pleasant," or "good." All of the descriptions hold an element of motivation—something that extends beyond the mundane, the everyday, the habitual. As we go through this book, I invite you to remember this. When you explore your own definition of desire, consider how that may (or may not) play into your description and ultimately your erotic template.

The Erotic Equation

One of the world's most insightful sexologists, Jack Morin, PhD, describes the visceral nature of desire through something he calls "the erotic equation." In his earth-shattering book *The Erotic Mind*,[1] Morin claims the erotic equation lies at the heart of desire and meaningful, fulfilling sex:

Attraction + Obstacles = Excitement

Morin's insightful revelation reminds us that desire is not simple and straightforward. Nor is it always pleasant. There is an element of tension to it for many of us, and sometimes it is this tension that causes us discomfort while simultaneously being incredibly appealing. This is partly why the first flush of a new relationship is so exciting—the object of our desire is not yet fully ours. We are excited by their presence but also unsure how long we will have them, where the relationship will go, or if they will stick around. We go out of our way to look good and smell good for them. We invest our own energy in making a good impression. The uneasiness between us is both terrifying and exciting. Hello, Desire!

Paying attention, remembering significant facts or events, taking care and showing enthusiasm are all indicators of a robust fascination and are often very present at the start of a new relationship. That element of excitement and attraction, coupled with the insecurity or instability of the relationship's future, combines to make a heady cocktail of lust and intrigue for many of us. Our partner is new and fascinating, and we revel in getting to know more about them. Their mere presence makes us feel a variety of feelings that we are *sure* come from the magical chemistry between us.

And in many ways, this is true. Our brains go into overdrive, producing an intoxicating elixir of chemicals that literally drive us wild. We long to get our hands on each other and we look forward to the next time we can be alone together.

But the difficulty for us is that we can't keep having first dates with the same person forever. Others seem to prefer a never-ending cycle of first dates with lots of people that often go nowhere, because the thrill of the chase is, for some, more attractive than the stability of a relationship or the promise of intimacy.

Couples in therapy often reminisce about the first six to twelve months, when their relationship was at its hottest. There was an erotic current between them that waned over time. While they recognize that this is "normal," they also long for that spark, often speaking of it as if it were something that happened to them rather than something they co-created between them.

The crucial "obstacle" of the unknown, the distance, the longing in Morin's equation, disappears when we fall into habits of established coupledom. We feel secure in our relationship. We've considered future plans, maybe moved in together, maybe bought property, or discussed starting a family. They've seen us in the morning, smelled our morning breath and our farts. The rawness of who we *really* are has been revealed. It feels like there's nothing else to discover. During this time, sex (sometimes) becomes mechanical or obligatory and we don't invest as much energy in wooing our lover. We already have them; we feel close and loved. It's secure and it's intimate, but often this comes at the cost of the excitement we also seek. For many of us, eroticism is the space between two parts of ourselves: our vulnerability and our excitement. This tension is the grain of sand that creates the pearl we call desire.

Renowned therapist Esther Perel also speaks of the chasm between our wish for security and our hunger for excitement. The erotic equation seems to be the answer to our problems, but she acknowledges that knowing this is one thing, while what do we do about it is a whole other dynamic. Through this book we will come back to this quandary in many ways, time and time again.

While Morin's work focuses on the nature of erotic fantasies, which we'll explore more in chapter 12, his insights help us better understand where our desires are located and how to activate them even in long-term partnerships. As someone who enjoys ideas immensely, I think it's helpful to have a robust vocabulary when exploring sex and desire. When we are able to describe in rich detail what we like or seek, we are better able to understand that and describe it to ourselves and eventually our partners.

For some people, however, words do not come easily. For them, desire is often something experienced viscerally, perhaps emotionally, more than simply as an idea. In many ways, desire is an *idea* that transforms into both a feeling and a sensation. Desire requires us to engage mentally, physically, and emotionally. This is special. Few of life's tasks require this, and this is also what makes it more complicated.

What's Love Got to Do with It?

Desire is often discussed in the context of intimate ongoing relationships and marriages. For many people, desire is synonymous with romantic love. One thing that desire and romantic love have in common is they are both difficult to define, highly controversial, and can be all-consuming.

Romantic love as we know it today in the West is, according to some, a relatively new concept in the history of the human species. Author C. S. Lewis suggests in *The Allegory of Love*[2] that its origins are transcendental in nature and were derived during medieval times, stemming from the notion of "courtly love" that was inspired by poets of the past and bestowed upon knights and damsels of France in the eleventh century. But this romantic all-consuming love was never intended to be consummated, nor to form the foundation of a lifelong partnership. While previous cultures and societies made reference to love—poets Rumi and Ovid spoke of its appeal and the story of Isis and Osiris was recorded more than three thousand years ago in ancient Egypt—romantic love, in the way Westerners refer to it now, as a basis for marriage and a pair-bonded monogamous relationship, is relatively modern. Love, it is suggested, is designed to transform, to inspire, and to revere. It was never intended to be sullied with such base notions as sex and lust. According to historian Simon May, "a philosophy of love, so this view goes, is either futile (love cannot be defined) or self-defeating (to define it is to degrade it)".[3]

Plato spoke of love as a guide to behaving with honor. It was not a lustful endeavor but rather a love between men that had neither to do with sex nor sexuality. It is from Plato's name that we derive the word "platonic," describing a connection based on honor rather than desire, implying that the two were mutually exclusive.

The most referenced document that illustrates the written origins of romantic love is the Old Testament's Song of Songs. However, while the text describes something whimsical and otherworldly in its appreciation of physicality and beauty, it does not necessarily describe love in detail, as distinct from an appreciation of physical form—something we associate with desire.

Despite this uncertain history, the rise of romantic love is one of the central tenets of connection and life's meaning within the Western psyche. Romantic love is revered as an essential ingredient to a fulfilled life. Pop culture would have us believe that without romantic love fulfilment is doomed. Books dedicated entirely to the notion of romantic love exist in abundance, form their own genre, and are marketed primarily at cis, heterosexual women. In popular and social media, celebrations of romantic love are everywhere: from human interest stories and status updates to the subject of clinical studies, films, and pop music.

Social historian Stephanie Coontz tells that the notions we have of love and indeed marriage today are grossly unrealistic. She asserts that for most of history, the notion of choosing a partner "on the basis of something as fragile and irrational as love and then focus all their sexual, intimate, and altruistic desires on the resulting marriage" is a ridiculous notion.[4] Throughout history, people have fallen in love, but it was only in the 1800s that this became considered an inspiration for marriage.

Modern Western culture insists that you bond with one person and meld everything: families, sexuality, finances, children, burdens, personalities, and responsibilities. The expectation is that one person is able to offer you everything that, once upon a time, an entire community would have supplied. So how did such ideas become so intertwined?

"Limerence," as coined by psychologist Dorothy Tennov, is the process of recognizing another in such a way that brings both our *attention* and *attraction*. More colloquially we call it "falling in love." We catch ourselves thinking about them, daydreaming about them, and overlooking their potential faults because, as noted by Chaucer, love is blind.

Time for Reflection

What stories were you brought up with about love and marriage? That you would find "The One"? That there was only one? That love was effortless with the right person? How did you absorb this information? Was it from children's stories when you were very small?

For many of us the path to love and marriage was expected, in some cases, pre-determined, depending where and how we grew up. For others our love interest may have been taboo, especially if we are queer in some way, or from a culture that has struggled to embrace the vastness of human sexual diversity. Taking time to consider how romance culture has influenced your understanding of relationships helps you develop perspective and context for the values you hold about love and relationships today. Write down your earliest memories of learning about love and romance. Think about your experiences of love and romance as an adult? How similar are they to the ideas you were raised with? Do you know anyone with a relationship like what you were taught? If so, what evidence do you have that their relationship is as fabulous as it looks? Taking the time to write about this (or draw it if writing doesn't work for you) helps you experience how these ideas may have influenced your expectations of love and romance, too.

While cultural anthropologists have drawn a variety of conclusions about the origin and purpose of romantic love, it has been and remains to this day, something mysterious and often difficult to maintain over extended periods of time.

The relationship between romantic love and desire is the source of many a self-help book and was the central tenet of marriage counseling theory for much of the twentieth century. The idea that "love is enough" and "if you love someone just the right way, the sex will just come naturally" has been at the heart of romantic literature and romantic comedies alike. It's also been at the center of much of Western sex education, reminding us that sex without love is dangerous (especially if you're a woman). The billion-dollar self-help industries, and more recently the "wellness" industries, have carried on the crusade to fuse love and desire firmly in the psyche of the Western consumer. The implication is that love will conquer all—even the Beatles told us "All You Need Is Love." But for many of us, love is simply not the path to desire. Nor is it enough.

Now, I don't want to rain on anyone's parade here. Challenging romantic love is a thorny issue. After all, people make huge life decisions based on this process—I'm not here to unravel it. I am interested, though, in inspiring an exploration of these ideas. Maybe through what we discover, we can learn more about ourselves and ultimately what our desires are.

Something that confuses many people I work with is why the feelings of love they have for their partner are more consistent than their feelings of desire for them. While the two tend to be lumped together, deeper exploration often reveals that they are not at all the same thing. This explains why so many people wonder if their long-term relationships are sustainable when their desire has waned: if losing the desire for sex means they simply do not love their partner anymore.

Case Study: Rhiannon
Rhiannon was at the end of her rope when she came to see me.

"What is wrong with me?" she asked rhetorically. She stretched her long arms out across the arm rest of the chair and looked wistfully out the window.

"Everyone tells me how lucky I am. I have a great partner and a gorgeous daughter . . . but I feel so empty inside. I feel . . . well, nothing."

Rhiannon's situation is common among many of the women I work with. What started out as a great thing slowly loses its gloss over time. It's not a question of losing her love for her family, but a question of finding herself.

"You know, I used to love sex. I *loved* it. I did it all. I was wild. When my husband Alex and I first got together, we'd really get into it. With each other, with others. We'd go to swinger parties and he loved watching me with other guys. I loved it too. But we were both drinking a lot then. It was fun but we knew it was unstable, so we gave up the booze completely when we found out I was pregnant."

"So that was around the same time that you started to notice a drop in your desire?" I asked.

"Well, yes, but its more than that. I actually think I was always like this. The alcohol gave me confidence"

I was curious; the confidence for *what?* I wondered.

"You mean it took your inhibitions away?" I inquired

"Yes, absolutely! I was unstoppable. But now, I barely tolerate sex with the lights on. We do it in the dark, or as dark as possible and as soon as it's over, I turn away from him. I get it over with because I love him and I don't want to lose him, but I hate that I don't enjoy it any more, even when I have orgasms, it's still not especially great."

Something about the performance versus the intimacy piqued my interest. Her desire used to be fueled by abandon, the temporary removal of social taboos seemed to increase the heat for her, but seemingly only in the presence of alcohol. And having kicked that habit after becoming a mother, Rhiannon was left with the cold reality that the desire she once embodied, the permission made possible by alcohol, was only accessible to her when she felt safe enough to drop her inhibitions, which, without booze, was infrequent.

"Sex now between just two of you, with no audience and no context sounds too intimate, . . . perhaps too close for you?" I wondered. I was curious about what she was feeling.

"It is!" she exclaimed. "It's really too much. Now I just don't want to be seen. Between him and my daughter, their need for attention is high. They both want to be near me all the time. I love them both so much. My God I am so lucky, but I just can't be that close all the time."

Like many women, the pressures of parenting, the obligation to be touched by kids and partners, takes its toll on their desire. Where touch used to be received as a gift, it now felt more like a loss. The very same action now meant something was being taken from her and left her feeling depleted. For Rhiannon, the party girl of her twenties got side-tracked to become the healthier, but equally distraught and frustrated mother, partner, and human in session with me today.

She went on to tell me about lovers from the past, all of whom offered *intrigue*. She felt like they took her on a journey.

"When I was twenty, I was seeing a guy in his forties. He was amazing. I was so excited by him and he taught me so much about sex. That really turned me on."

"Who else?" I asked

"My first boyfriend was really romantic. We were in high school and I was totally head over heels for him too."

"What did you like about these two guys especially?" I asked.

She pondered a moment and after some time she realized they both, along with her husband, in the beginning, and her time with the swinger community, were all about lifting her out of her daily life. For her, it wasn't so much about the excitement as it was about being centered, like *she really mattered* to them. These practices and these men at one time made her feel *special*—not just wanted. She felt *wanted* now, but with the demands on her, she no longer feels *special*. This insight was a crucial distinction for her erotic template.

For Rhiannon, her love was never questioned, nor was the quality of the sex, but in knowing what brought her desire to life, she was better able to focus on it and understand how to communicate it to her husband without him feeling he was doing something wrong or that she was defective. In Rhiannon's case, she was a classic example of love in abundance, but none of the ingredients to ignite her desire.

If you were to think about how you like sex to make you feel, what might it be? There are of course multiple answers and, in Rhiannon's case, feeling *special* was particularly important. One key ingredient of her erotic template is the longing to feel special.

So, let's take a closer look at what desire means—to you personally.

Meeting Desire

I like to describe *love* and *desire* like chocolate and red wine. (Feel free to substitute other delicious morsels here if you are a non-drinker or not into chocolate.) They can and do go together as if they were made for each other, but they can also be enjoyed alone. They can also be the cause of pain and distress if they are not respected and taken care of. Too much or too often can be destructive, and too little or too infrequent can leave you longing.

You can survive and live perfectly well without chocolate and red wine. You can love someone with all your heart and not desire them. You can desire someone you know isn't good for you, have never met, or that you met only five minutes ago. Just like we saw with Rhiannon, her desire became accessible when her inhibitions were reduced and when she felt special. It's hard to say for her which came first, whether feeling special gave her permission to let go, or whether letting go gave her the thrill of feeling special, but either way, what brought her to my office and what brings many to sex therapy globally, is a longing to return to what was once alive and has been lost, if it ever was there.

I want to emphasize, again, the importance of developing a vocabulary around desire. Desire is something that is often kept in the dark and associated with shame and guilt. Like Rhiannon she felt terribly guilty for not desiring her husband the way she used to even though there was no doubt she loved him. The more we can shed light on what we want sex to offer us, the more likely we are to be able to see it and find ways to bring it into our lives in ways that are fulfilling and helpful to us. By identifying and naming our feelings and ideas about desire, we gain more power in our relationship with them.

This activity is designed to get you engaging with the concepts of love and desire in ways that are reflective, gentle, and insightful. Don't go racing ahead. Just work through the pages, bit by bit.

Exploring Love and Desire

Open your note book to a new page and divide it into two columns. Mark one column "Love" and the other "Desire." As a prompt, write all the words you associate with love under the "Love" column and likewise with desire:

- When I think about "love" these words come to mind . . .
- When I think about "desire" these words come to mind . . .

If writing is not your thing, drawing is also welcome.

- What (if anything) do these groups of words have in common? (Look for themes, symbols, feelings, sensation, etc, not linguistic features.)
- What distinguishes love from desire based on the map you have drafted?
- Consider the *tone* of the words—are they urgent or gentle?
- Are they based in the senses (physical) or in fantasies / the imagination (psychological / emotional)?
- How does it feel to look at these words and sit with them?

- What's happening in your body right now?
- How are you breathing?
- How easy is it to concentrate right now?
- Do you need a break? Take one!
- What emotions are present? These may be comfortable emotions like *peace* or *relief*, or they may be feelings of *confusion*, *restlessness*, or *anxiety*. All are welcome and normal.

As far as possible, try not to judge them. Simply acknowledge them and write them in your note book without trying to change or supress them. Hold onto them as we'll be coming back to these later on when formulating more of your erotic template. Their presence is a valuable tool in understanding your historic and present relationship with desire and love.

This practice may be a little surprising for you, especially if you have never considered the differences before. Staying with the inquiry is helpful to gain the skills you need to learn more about the foundations of your erotic template as we move forward.

If this is the first time you have considered the distinction between *love* and *desire*, allow yourself time to absorb this new knowledge. See where it leads you. It might be liberating. It might be challenging. It might be old news. No matter what, getting used to self-reflection to solve erotic quandaries is going to be a useful skill for the rest of your life.

It can be good to revisit this activity from time to time, as it allows you to reflect on what your ideas and also your feelings about love and desire are, and how they change over time and as you travel through this book.

What Do Desire and Love Mean to You?

Consider these prompts and complete the sentence in a way that feels right for you.

Desire
- Desire is . . .
- Desire feels like . . .

- As a young person I was brought up to believe / I believed desire was . . .
- In my community / family / relationship desire is considered to be . . .
- When I hear the word "desire," I think of . . .
- If desire were a color, it would be . . .
- If I could taste desire, it would taste like . . .
- If I could smell desire, it would smell like . . .
- If I could touch desire, it would feel like . . .
- I physically feel desire in / on my . . .
- When I talk about desire, I feel . . .
- I can talk about desire with . . .
- My strongest experience of desire to date is / was / could be . . .

Love
- Love is . . .
- Love feels like . . .
- As a young person I was brought up to believe / I believed love was . . .
- In my community / family / relationship love is considered . . .
- When I hear the word "love," I think of . . .
- If love were a color, it would be . . .
- If I could taste love, it would taste like . . .
- If I could smell love, it would smell like . . .
- If I could touch love, it would feel like . . .
- I physically feel love in / on my . . .
- When I talk about love, I feel . . .
- I can talk about love with . . .
- My strongest experience of love to date is / was / could be . . .

Were there any surprises in these answers? Any that were especially difficult? Or easy? Any that you especially enjoyed? Or especially disliked?

Practicing noticing your feelings and responses to things without shutting them out is a powerful skill to cultivate. Curiosity about yourself and others is a valuable tool in discovering desire, and one we'll explore more in chapter 7.

Reflecting on What Desire and Love Mean and Feel like to You

Leave this reflection exercise for a day or two and return to it later. It's vital that you progress slowly and comfortably with these exploratory processes. By allowing ourselves time to adjust to new ideas, experiences, and ways of being, we allow our minds and bodies time to adjust to these new possibilities. We are digging through many decades of conditioning. Coming to understand new ways of being must be done gently and with care—both for ourselves and for those who may be affected by our discoveries. We are not ripping down old structures, merely excavating their foundations to see what we can find and maybe rebuild.

When you are ready, take a look at your responses to the questions above.

Are you surprised by anything? Notice how the language you use to discuss love and the language you use to discuss desire may be similar, yet may also be different.

Responses from Others

SARTIA: I was amazed at how different my lists of words were when I looked at them. The words I used to describe desire had a feeling of intensity about them while the words I used to describe love had a calm feeling. I was surprised because like so many others I had thought that love would lead to desire, but when I stop to think about it, the way I relate to these things is really quite different—intense and not intense. Desire feels hot and nearly a little anxiety-inducing, there's a pressure there somehow—but love feels more relaxed, accepting, and easy—for me anyhow.

MARK: Desire for me feels guilty. I have never told anyone about my desires because I feel ashamed of them. I don't think I could find anyone who could want to act on them with me, sometimes I don't know if I want to either. But I know what gets me turned on and I don't like that that's how it is. I wish I was desiring of other things. I don't like to talk about it—except here in therapy. I don't *like* it here either, but I do it.

TARA: I was surprised how reflecting on desire made me feel sad. Not sad because I think it's bad, but sad because I used to feel it and I don't feel it anymore. It feels like something I used to have, but now, responsibility has taken over and life is just not as fun as it used to be. I guess I am not desiring of much anymore. But I would like to be again.

CLARE: My response to desire feels naughty, in a fun way. It's like I can really let myself go when I think about what desire means to me. Sometimes among my friends we talk about our escapades and we sound traditionally like men. We are proud of our activities and sometimes challenge each other to go further. But on other days I reflect on this and I start to feel ashamed, I imagine that other women are not like me, like us—and maybe there is something wrong with me. I feel guilty and ashamed, but then I let it wash over me and I feel inspired again. It's like a dance I am getting used to. When I am feeling good about myself it feels OK, but if I start feeling vulnerable, I can really talk myself down. I am learning its patterns now and I am practicing not judging myself for the ideas and feelings that I have. It's hard. But I keep practicing.

Based on these reflections and your own, in what ways would you say love and desire are different? What different feelings, emotions, ideas, and sensations do they bring up for you? What does this context suggest for you about how love and desire function in your life?

ROY: We got married in India and then moved to Australia where we live a very non-traditional lifestyle. In India we were in a pretty liberal community but, even still, the social pressures to have a physical relationship are pretty strong if you are married. I really love my wife but the sex between us is dismal. Love makes me feel obligated to not stray and sometimes this makes me sad. The desire part of me wants to just leave but I stay because I love her and I learned that I associate love with obligation. I'm not a very traditional person, but I do believe in integrity—so I stay even though it's difficult.

ADELE: When I think about love I think about connection. I think about feeling safe and held and taken care of. I think about spending lazy Sundays on the couch together, or gardening together, or talking about our plans for the future together. I imagine feeling understood. It feels nice and comforting. I guess if love were a food, it would be chicken soup. It heals everything. I am much more familiar with love than desire and I didn't realize this until just now. Love feels safe and familiar—desire feels distant, foreign—to me anyway.

Taking the time to reflect on desire and how we relate to it in contrast with love helps us get closer to it, especially if we were raised with them fused together. For most of us desire was something we absorbed by osmosis from the cultures around us, the communities we inhabit, and, perhaps, the sex education we received. From the examples above, we see that desire and love do create different feelings for people, but often feelings we don't expect, like sadness or loneliness on the one hand, or passion and pleasure on another, and sometimes all of them at once. Moving forward, we'll learn more about what these paradoxes mean, how they show up in our lives, and how to work *with* them to create the desire and connections we hope for from sex. No matter how you come to conceptualize desire, know that it is open to change, depending upon how you change and learn more about yourself. In the next chapter we will look at some of the most common yet destructive myths about desire that trip people up in their quest for passion. We'll consider how we got to be so removed from the complexity of sex and relationships, who benefits from keeping us in the dark, and what we can do to start shedding more light on our understandings and investigations.

CHAPTER 4

Desire Myths

It's easier to fool people than to convince them that they have been fooled.

—(maybe) Mark Twain

In the last chapter we looked at the difference between romantic love and sexual desire and how helpful (or unhelpful) it is to lump the two together. We considered how desire can often bring up complicated feelings, that have less to do with pleasure and more to do with our sense of belonging—to ourselves and to our relationships. Indeed, desire is a fraught experience for so many of us and is likely what brought you to this book in the first place. In this chapter, we get clinical as we drop deeper into sexual desire to learn some of the common myths we mistake for facts, and again consider their effect and influence in our lives, our choices in sex, and the assumptions we make about ourselves and our partners as sexual beings. Toward the end, things get a little nerdy but bear with it. The clinical theories offer some useful context into how modern desire research has evolved in contrast with our cultural narratives about sex being easy.

When you recall your own experiences of learning about sex, pleasure, and desire, consider how much helpful information you received. How much of the information you have about sex actually addresses the *real* reasons people have sex, how they do it and what they do? For many of us, sex education was rudimentary at best—if it existed at all. For a lot of us, there were, and are, a lot of gaps to fill. And as we go through life, having relationships and sexual experiences, we tend to draw conclusions based on minimal information. There is a lack of permission to seek out new knowledge or explore new ways of being, simply because there is an element of shame in doing so. To *not know* these things as an adult implies that we are somehow defective. To struggle with sex and the pleasure of relationships means we have lost our way.

But, if we were never taught to value such information:

- How are we able to create and sustain useful self-inquiry about desire?
- How are we able to initiate conversations about desire?
- Are we even allowed to have conversations about our desires?
- How do we allow ourselves to admit we don't know stuff without risking the wash of shame associated with talking about sex?

This will all be addressed as you build your erotic template. But when certain topics are taboo, or we are not allowed to speak, our silence creates a veneer of shame. Within this shame, misinformation flourishes, because it doesn't occur to us there is another way through.

But I want to again reiterate to you, there *are* other ways of relating to sex and pleasure. Seeking knowledge is perfectly acceptable and, ultimately, essential.

Myths arise and flourish when education, reflection, and inquiry are not encouraged. We don't realize their effects on our pleasure and experiences. We doubt ourselves because we are more accustomed to understanding our sexual experiences through cultural mythology of what is "normal," than we are to understanding our very own lived experience. But the truth is, despite many studies done over fifty years on what constitutes normal sex (in the West, at least), the results are inconclusive. In other words, no one can really say what, exactly, "normal" sex is.

Time for Reflection

Most of us were taught that sex was natural and for making babies. But for most of us, that's not really why we do it, nor does it come to us so easily at all. Yet, for most of us, we can identify those two myths embedded in our earliest awareness of sex education. What were some other beliefs about sex you grew up with? Write them in your notebook.

For example:

- Did your parents talk about sex at home? When they did, were they comfortable doing so?
- When did you discover sex was even a thing? How old were you?
- You were likely taught that sex was between a man and woman and that it always involved penis-in-vagina sex. Why do you think this is the way sex was taught, given that people experience sex in so many varied ways?
- If your introduction to sex was more open, do you remember learning explicitly about pleasure? Your own? Other people's? Was it valued? Or was it swept under the rug?

The reason for this is simple. Sexuality is fluid, changeable, and dependent on a variety of cultural, emotional, physiological, mental, relational, and educational contexts and is affected by gender, race, mobility, ability, age, affluence, privilege, identity, and much more. What you enjoyed, were able to do, or even interested in at eighteen is unlikely to be what you experience now, nor is it what you will experience twenty, thirty, or fifty years from now. For some this may be disappointing; for others a relief. Our relationship with sex and pleasure changes over our lifetime, yet few of us take the time to consider its relevance or how this affects our connection with sex in the present. In this sense, sexual energy is more like water than fixed like stone. It fluctuates according to the environment it's in. It heats up. It cools down. Sometimes it freezes and sometimes it dries up, but never completely—even if it feels like that. And like water, it gets in everywhere. Wherever there's an opening (no pun intended) there's an opportunity for water to get in. Just like the influence of the moon on oceans, the influence on your sexual energy and incentive is you. All of you. Your relationships, your lovers, your upbringing, your history, your experiences, your beliefs, your values, your identity, your environment, and, most of all, your sex education.

What's Sex Education Got to Do with It?

Sex education is for everyone, especially for those whose sex education was lacking in complexity, variety, and, essentially, truth (which, let's face it, is most of us).

Sexology is still a very new field of study and while a study of sexual cultures among Western heterosexuals might suggest a certain level of frequently occurring assumptions, studies conducted on sexual practices of women, men, and non-binary people of varied orientations in other parts of the world may yield vastly different results. This is because human sexuality is borne of culture, not solely biology. What is considered "normal" in one sexual culture is not necessarily normal in another.

For example, heterosexuals are not accustomed to questioning sex and sexuality because they are accustomed to being the default against which normal is measured. It is assumed that they will all have penis-in-vagina (PIV) sex and they will like it, in much the same way that it is assumed that all gay men enjoy anal sex and that all lesbians enjoy oral sex. We tend to not think about the sex lives and pleasure of gender-diverse people beyond how they appeal to cis people, rather than how they experience themselves as agents of their own desire and pleasure. But the truth is that what we enjoy in bed and how we identify are not always the same thing. Just because you like eating carrots, doesn't make you a vegetarian!

A perfect example of this is penis-in-vagina intercourse. Many heterosexuals are expected to engage in PIV intercourse with little reflection on why it has become the default sexual practice for heterosexuals. When I ask heterosexuals why they think this is the case, they are often surprised at my line of questioning, but even more surprised by their own response. Most of the time, they are not really sure why they are doing it, or why sex without it, often referred to as "foreplay," is considered a lesser form of sex. Foreplay suggests there is a grander, superior act coming; foreplay is merely a precursor to the "main event." But mysteriously, no one knows why we see it this way. It's just a given.

When pushed further, many heterosexual cis men will say PIV feels good (which is perfectly fine). But this all comes tumbling down when they struggle to get or sustain erections or when they ejaculate too quickly. Then intercourse is off the menu—temporarily at least. It no longer feels good but is instead a source of shame and anxiety. The one thing straight cis men have been told to invest their sexual confidence in, is now no longer accessible to them. They will do anything to get back to that feeling of "being normal," because that's simply what heterosexuals are expected to do.

Heterosexual women engage in PIV intercourse for even less-established reasons than men. Many say it feels "good" (many also say it feels "boring" or even "painful"), but it is not the kind of "good" that creates an orgasm for most. For the vast majority of heterosexual women who say that PIV sex is "good," it is experienced more as psychologically arousing than physiologically arousing, but few of our cultural discussions reflect this phenomenon. Yet both they and their male partners persevere with PIV sex because, between heterosexuals, PIV is sacred. Or rather, it's "normal." Overwhelmingly, in my experience many people just want to be "normal," whether it feels good and brings pleasure or not. In many cases, being "normal" is more important than feeling good. Many of us stick with the script because it simply doesn't occur to us that there might be something else we could do that would bring greater satisfaction. People engage in sex practices because they think they are:

- normal,
- what's expected, and / or
- what everyone else is doing

rather than because they actually have a personal reason for doing so.

Busting through the Barriers of Normal

As we have discovered, so much of what people struggle with regarding sex and their desire, or lack of desire, for it is based on feelings of inadequacy regarding how they perceive themselves or how they will be perceived by their lovers or partners. Will they still be seen as acceptable by those who matter?

For example, straight cis men can enjoy receiving penetration and gay men can find themselves attracted to hetero porn and conservatives can find themselves wanting to explore rough sex and bondage. Then, just when you thought it was settled, that can all change at any moment. All this can be a source of inquiry for many people.

I meet a lot of self-identified "queer" women who want to know more about their desires. A lot of straight cis women who wonder why they don't enjoy intercourse. A lot of gay, bi, and straight cis men who have trouble understanding why their erections are unreliable or why blow jobs feel boring. Others want to know what their fantasies mean, while some are questioning gender and gender roles, and a lot of people want to talk about porn and how they feel about what they like and don't like to watch. Many want to know what to be aware of in an open relationship and a lot want to keep it just between them and their one beloved, while others want to know how to reconcile their sexual interests and their religious beliefs.

You can see why a "one size fits all" approach to sex just doesn't work.

The trouble is that, for a lot of people, sex is not nearly as fulfilling as it could be because most of us simply do not have the tools to explore and communicate it. If you didn't learn it at school, haven't really considered your erotic motivations that much, and you haven't experimented a lot (or you have experimented but have come up against a road block), this is exactly where changing and expanding your thinking about sex can really help if you're struggling with mismatched libido or low desire.

Case Study: Shona and Maze

Shona and Maze, two queer women, were in a rut. Both of them accomplished professionals in their field, worked long hours, and had been living together for the better part of their eight-year relationship. Sex between them was never really "hot," which was OK but, over time, Shona became increasingly resentful of Maze's lack of enthusiasm. Maze never initiated sex and Shona was angry. By the time I saw them, Shona had started to wonder if perhaps Maze may be asexual. Initially Maze reached out to me alone, explaining that Shona was angry at her for not liking sex. Certainly, that was Maze's understanding. But when I finally met with Shona it turned out that she was not mad at Maze for *not liking* sex, but for ignoring the issue of sex between them and doing it every time Shona raised it. For Shona, it was like she was talking and the mic was off; over time it came to pass that she shutdown, became resentful, and they were considering separation. After further inquiry between them, Maze confirmed she was not asexual, but had certainly grown up feeling awkward about sex with little knowledge of what people did or how to process the feelings that accompanied it. In her Catholic family, sex was neither spoken of nor encouraged, and if anything Maze recalled how her mother actively discouraged her from having a relationship with her body at all. For Maze, her body felt strange, aloof, and when in the early part of their relationship Shona tried to access it, Maze would check out, feeling very little and not responding much to touch nor discussion. Maze shared with me that when they did have sex, Shona often wanted for sex to happen toward her but she'd neglect to return the favor to Maze. Maze really wanted Shona to understand it wasn't that she didn't *like* sex, it was that she was stuck in a pattern of confusion around pleasure, around her body, and she really wanted Shona to touch her back, but didn't know how to express it because, until then, she'd never really realized she was allowed to. For Shona, the lack of communication, Maze's difficulty remaining present during sex and the lack of frequency made her feel rejected. Over time Maze recognized she had a choice. The myths she'd inherited about sex from her family and community were not true. She really needed to lift her game and start working more on being present with her own body and responding to Shona's requests, at least with acknowledgment rather than leaving Shona hanging, feeling unheard. Maze finally understood that waiting for the mood to strike, and for her to magically have the sexual confidence she dreamed of, wouldn't just fall from the sky. That if she really wanted to stay with Shona, she'd have to learn more about her own body, how to ask for what she wanted and how to stay present to her feelings when arousal started to rise within her. For Maze this was ground breaking. All her life she'd assumed sex was natural. That everyone was having great sex except her, not because she'd never learned, but because she was defective. The good news was that she'd found a way through the dilemma. The even better news was that she discovered she'd had the tools all along. The final part was busting the myths that were holding her back from putting the tools to use.

Top Five Myths

Like Maze, many people believe myths about sex and desire that have a catastrophic effect on their relationships. Some of these might be very familiar to you, others might not be, but if you grew up in the West, it's likely they've been in your orbit too.

1. Frequency of Sex

How many times have you seen a segment on a TV show that begins discussions of sex with a decimal number of how many times a week couples around the world are "doing it"? This is a phrase and an idea that we use to gauge how our libido matches up to other people's. We compare ourselves to others, even though the reality is we have no idea how other people have sex nor whether they're even enjoying it, no matter how often they're doing it.

Somehow we have managed to equate frequency with quality and, instead of wondering what we are getting out of it or what purpose it serves, we are spending a lot more time fretting about:

How many times a week should we be doing it?

The problem is when we try to shoehorn ourselves into being "normal" regarding frequency, we take our attention away from the quality of the experience:

We want to be doing it two or three times a week.
We want to do it once a month.
We want to be doing it once every six months.

The truth is frequency doesn't matter much, unless, of course, it matters to you. If so, that's fine. It could be helpful to ask yourself:

What does frequency of sex represent to me / us?

Or even:

Why is frequency of sex important in this context?

- Does it mean you are more loved?
- More loving?
- Hotter?
- Your relationship is not falling apart?
- Or something else entirely?

The truth is it doesn't really matter *why* you want it more but rather that *you* know *what is motivating* the struggle for more, especially if you are dissatisfied with the frequency. If we don't reflect on this question, we can end up spending a lot of energy feeding anxiety rather than focusing on the very thing we want to get from sex in the first place.

So while the frequency question is a big one to start with, it's one that masks an even more important, or certainly more relevant, question that tends to be omitted from this conversation. The question is, of course, about *quality*:

How good should sex be when we have it?

This is not a question partners often discuss. What even constitutes "good"? (We'll get to that in chapter 7.) If you have decided that frequency is important to you, we can then look at it in a much broader context. Does increased frequency mean you're going to be having more sex because it's *better*? If you're having a high frequency of sex:

- Are you then also going to be focused on quality every time?
- Is that feasible for you?

- How will you manage that?
- When would be the right times to make that happen?

Remember that focusing on frequency is fine, except that we can get tricked into thinking that the more we do it the better off we are. And the truth is, that's not always the case. Research suggests that quality matters more.[1]

2. Sex Is Natural

When I suggest that the naturalness of sex is a myth, the responses I get are similar to those you might get when you tell a child Santa Claus isn't real and neither is the Easter Bunny nor the Tooth Fairy. People look forlorn, gutted, and even horrified. I have even had people on talkback radio get angry with me, insisting that sex *is* natural; it's evolution and that's how we came to be here!

That's all well and good, and certainly the premise of propagating the species may be natural, but that kind of "reproduction-style" sex has very little to do with pleasure, especially for women, gay men, lesbians, non-binary people, and all the others whose sexuality sits outside the reproduction versus pleasure square. That kind of quick, no-warm-up, just-get-the-seed-in-there style of sex just doesn't feel that good to most of us. Yet a lot of us, regardless of gender or orientation, are very invested in the "naturalness" of sex, and any idea that it's not, is not just abhorrent but downright misery-inducing. I get that, I really do, but let me explain what I mean.

Dr. Leonore Teifer is a psychiatrist and psychotherapist of phenomenal renown, based in New York City. Her thought-provoking book, *Sex Is Not a Natural Act*,[2] thoroughly critiques and dissects many of the assertions of early sexology, claiming that the biological imperatives proposed by clinical and medical sexology simply serve the needs of (heterosexual) men and only look at the physiological elements of sex while dismissing the emotional and cultural contexts in which they play out.

But if sex isn't *natural*, then what is it?

I'd argue that aspects of sex are natural, to a degree. What's natural about sex for a lot of us, but not all, is the urge. It's the *instinct*, it's *that* curiosity. You see it in small children and, to a lesser degree, in teenagers. When I say "small children," I'm not talking about a carnal, lusty urge or instinct. I don't necessarily think children have that. But what they *do* have is a playful inclination to seek pleasure that is physical, emotional, and, to a degree, sexual, but not necessarily erotic.

How many times have we found the toddler in our lives with their hand down their pants? And they think nothing of doing so. You've seen it—and most likely done it too, at that age. Watching very small children is a remarkable way to see the essence of the human condition in action, completely unfettered. They are pleasure-seeking machines who have yet to learn cultural and behavioral filters about what's OK and what's not. When people describe the naturalness of sex, they are in effect describing this *instinct*, rather than the crafted set of maneuvers we refer to when we discuss "sex" as adults.

Now, think about the first time that you had sex, whatever that means to you. How did that feel? Were you as graceful as a swan on an open lake at dusk, brimming with confidence, gliding across the erotic waters with absolutely no problems at all? Or were you a little bit more like a foal taking its first steps? I would suggest that most of us were probably in this latter category. For a lot of us, sex acts and their execution don't come naturally *at all*.

Sex is something we need to learn. Sex is an art, a craft, and like any good art or craft, it takes skill, repetition, and practice. Historically, there have been few places we can go to get this knowledge (these days there are increasingly more). For many of us the craft of sex is something we are no more gifted at expressing than drawing or macramé. We haven't practiced enough to make it something we have confidence in and knowledge of.

The bottom line is that we get misled into thinking that because sex is "natural," we should be able to download this information into our heads with little thought, regard, or effort. We are encouraged to believe its naturalness means we needn't invest too much attention or energy into it. Like the instinct to chew and swallow food, we simply should know how to do it.

But, using this same metaphor, just because we are able to chew and swallow, are we capable of creating Michelin-star meals? That kind of logic seems implausible. Yet we believe and even defend the idea that we don't need to learn about sex, it just happens. And when you love somebody enough, it just oozes out of you because . . . that's just how sex is.

Sadly, that's not true. Sex is something that we definitely need to practice. Just like being an artist, cook, or musician, you must practice your craft and learn new things and learn new ways of engaging with it in order to bring you and your partner(s) more pleasure. There's absolutely no shame in needing to polish our skills every now and again. Investing in learning how sex works for you is a really helpful thing to do.

3. Desire Is Natural

I'm hoping by now you're getting a sense of not only how pervasive the "natural" sex argument is but also how unhelpful it is. It's not that long ago that anything outside of "heterosexuality" and PIV sex was considered "unnatural." This was not only a moral justification but also a scientific justification that determined what kind of sex was and wasn't acceptable. In many parts of the world this is still a widely held belief, and one that destroys lives, relationships, and pleasure every single day. When it comes to sex, the truth is that the only thing that is natural is that it is experienced differently by everyone.

When people speak of desire being natural, they are often referring to a spontaneous urge, a feeling from within that manifests quite simply as a desire to engage in sex of some kind. And while this is indeed a real thing that many of us may have experienced, it's neither consistent nor reliable. Yet for many of us, it's the default template that determines whether or not we are willing to give ourselves over to an erotic experience.

For many of us, sex is far more complex than a basic A + B = C experience. The most common questions I am asked by couples in counseling sessions are:

Why aren't our libidos in sync?
Why isn't desire easy for me?
Why does my mind wander off during sex?
Why am I never in the mood?

The answer is that these are all perfectly natural variations of the myth that desire is natural. This myth expects us to believe, without a doubt, that *the physiological urge* toward sex, sometimes called *lust* or *horniness*, is the sole driver of the sexual experience, that it's effortless, and that without it we are simply not "in the mood" or able to enjoy ourselves.

As we will find out later, the idea of a "sex drive," that sex is a biological imperative for everyone, is false. We are going to find out that sex can be induced by biological incentives like lust and horniness, but it can also be induced by mental, emotional, and contextual ones. To consider this further, if there's nothing more to sex than carnal lust, why then are our collective ideas of love and sex so fundamentally linked? There is definitely a relationship between the two, but it is not as straightforward as we have been led to believe and, as we discovered in the previous chapter, it is infinitely more complex. If motivations other than physical were not part of desire, I propose that those inclined toward only the physical aspects of sex would be satisfied with solo masturbation and not bother partnering up, paying for sexual services, or bothering to seek sexual therapy when things "dried up."

The trouble is, many of us feel that the biological imperatives are more valuable, more real, or a more accurate representation of *authentic* desire or true lust. But our motivations for having sex come from a much broader variety of sources than simply a biological fix. While sexual activity and sexual satisfaction change what happens in our brains and vice versa (more on this in chapter 5), our reasons for engaging in sex vary widely, even within the same person at different times in our lives. This is perfectly normal. When we reflect on our own lives, we can see that our personal reasons for having sex are much more complex than simply a biological urge (something we will go into more in chapter 6). While at times horniness may be a driver, it's neither constant nor is it something we can anticipate being reliable or regular.

The notion that we should all want sex in the same way with the same frequency as a measure of a "healthy" relationship is also untrue. So is the idea that sexual desire for a partner is an accurate gauge of how much we love them. There are countless people on the planet who find desire for someone they love mind-bogglingly difficult, but feel rampant desire for someone they glimpsed on a train. As we explored in chapter 3, love and desire are fundamentally different yet deliciously complementary things, but allowing ourselves to get stuck in the need for them to be the same is as unhelpful as it is uninformed.

4. Desire Is Essential to Good Sex
This is another great myth, and one that many of us have a fundamental investment in. But where did we learn that this was how it was supposed to be? Who told us this? Did we somehow absorb the idea by osmosis?

The reality is that sex is not so black and white. Sex is a paradox, and desire is paradoxical by association. We feel things that contrast with what we're thinking. We experience something physiologically that contrasts with what our mind is doing. This is all part of the richness of desire. Part of this is recognizing that thought, feeling, sensation, and experience are all important but distinct aspects of human sexual response.

Let's take a moment to look at a couple of influential and important clinical models of desire. The first one is the infamous "Human Sexual Response" model posited by Masters and Johnson in 1966 (see figure 4.1).[3]

Some of you may be familiar with Masters and Johnson. The TV series *Masters of Sex* that was a hit several years ago was all about William Masters and Virginia Johnson. They were sexologists during the 1950s and 1960s—incredibly progressive at the time and, in many ways, even now. A lot of the work that people are doing in the field of sexology now is based on the research that Masters and Johnson did all those years ago. Some of the research has progressed since then. And, sadly, some of it hasn't.

According to Masters and Johnson, sex starts with excitement. For many of us, excitement in a sexual sense is synonymous with desire—getting in the mood, feeling frisky, feeling horny, feeling up-for-it, or DTF. According to this model, being "in the mood" is implied by the excitement phase and, thus, must be present for sex to take place. (Bear in mind that when Masters and Johnson refer to sex, they are essentially referring to sex that involves genitals—primarily PIV. They don't reference sex that involves clitorises, soft penises, anuses, or mouths, and certainly not sex that doesn't involve genitals.)

Next, we are introduced to the idea of the plateau stage. During and slightly after the excitement stage comes the engorgement of genital tissue. During the plateau stage we (might):

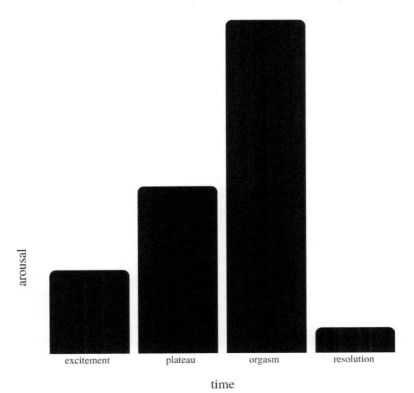

Figure 4.1. Masters and Johnson Model of Human Sexual Response, 1966.
Source: W. Masters and V Johnson. 1966. Human Sexual Response. Little, Brown and Company, p. 5.

- get and sustain an erection;
- get a swollen vulva;
- get and sustain wet labia and vagina;
- get dilation of the pupils; and/or
- get a flush around the chest.

We reach a plateau where this continues and it might continue for . . . well, who knows? Let's say "some time." Perhaps two minutes, or twenty minutes, or an hour. We sustain the physiological presence of a flushed sensation, a rich, embodied eroticism that is swollen, wet, and thick.

Then, according to Masters and Johnson, we have a KAPOW moment—an orgasm. This is a contentious and difficult issue, particularly, but not exclusively, for a lot of women and people with vulvas. However, the belief used to be that this happened for everyone, regardless of sexual style, orientation, or preferred practice. Furthermore, that the orgasm *was essential* to "real sex." After that comes the resolution stage, where we relax, happy orgasm chemicals are released, and our bodies return to normal.

While this model is indeed robust and was certainly a groundbreaking approach to sex and the field of sexology in general, we have since learned to consider new and more comprehensive ways of understanding how sex works. We now acknowledge that there is much more to great sex than simply physiological processes.

Although the Masters and Johnson model is still a default for many, especially in the medical professions, we now know that it is missing the emotional and psychological components of sex that also have an enormous impact on our sexual well-being. Reducing sex to a simple set of maneuvers left simply up to chance reduces our understanding of its potential and how to harness it for our own benefit.

We are doing ourselves a disservice if we omit the fact that sex is also emotional and psychological, regardless of our gender, orientation, or relationship status. As mentioned previously, if it were simply physical, we would be satisfied with masturbation, but many of us have a longing for something deeper and richer. (For the record, masturbation is fine. In fact, it's fabulous. It serves its purpose and it's a wonderful learning tool and experience all by itself, as you will discover if you haven't already.) But there is also something about partnered sex and our engagement with our own bodies in tandem with another that is more than simply "getting off."

In 2001, more than thirty years later, the Canadian sex professor and researcher Rosemary Basson proposed an alternative system called the Human Sexual Response Cycle (see figure 4.2).[4]

First of all, it's obvious that this is not a linear graph with a peak and a drop. This is a circle. That means there is no official starting point, so we can begin anywhere in the circle that we like. This is a dramatically different model than the previous. Not only is it circular, suggesting that human sexuality is more of a cycle than a one-way,

Basson's Human Sex Response Cycle: Circular Model. 2001

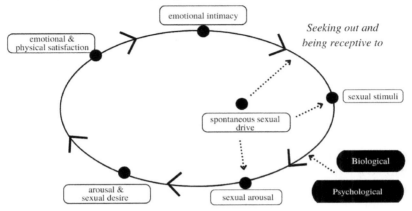

Figure 4.2. Basson's Human Sex Response Cycle: Circular Model.
Source: Rosemary Basson, "Human Sex Response Cycles," *Journal of Sex and Marital Therapy*
(2001): 33–43.

linear experience, but it also suggests that *desire does not have to pre-cede* arousal. In fact, it emphasizes a variety of possibilities, including the importance of mental and emotional cues, which the Masters and Johnson model neglects.

This leads us, then, to the next question: How are desire and arousal different? And does it matter? Briefly speaking, arousal is the physiological component of sexual excitement—the swelling, the engorgement, the erection, the lubrication, the flush, the increased heart rate. Arousal, by definition, is the purely physical. Desire, on the other hand, is the psychological and emotional components interacting with the biochemical components to create the sensation of being in-the-mood, feeling horny, feeling lusty, feeling engaged on a level greater than simply physical.

The Masters and Johnson model implies that arousal and desire come together in that first peak and that without them we cannot approach the "plateau." Criticism of this model emerged in the 1970s led by Helen Singer Kaplan[5] who created the Triphasic Model—where the concept of *sexual desire followed by arousal then orgasm* was first brought into view among clinicians. However, it wasn't until the 1990s that desire was to be explored in any way that involved emotions or other inhibitory factors (more on that in the next chapter), which make desire problematic. In 2000, there was a shift to a more holistic understanding of human sexual response that incorporated not only desire, arousal, and inhibitions but also emotions and contexts that allow sex to flourish. The main criticisms of the Masters and Johnson linear model are that it neither addresses the reasons for sex nor does it consider the complexity or variety of sexual experiences many of us have through the course of our life. In contrast, the Basson model suggests that sexual connection can start anywhere within the circle, and needn't even begin with desire. Our reasons may be more emotional than carnal (longing for or wanting connection and intimacy) or they can be a response to sexual stimuli (sexting, dirty talk, flirting, erotic images or porn, watching a partner undress or masturbate) or other psychological or contextual factors. Basson does not downplay biological influences or spontaneous impulses, she simply suggests that there's more going on than merely orgasm alone. In essence, this model identifies that people have a variety of reasons and motivations for having sex and that desire is not necessarily the primary one.

What makes this model unique is that it was the first time a model of sexuality suggested that arousal can precede desire. This is a revolutionary perspective and is extremely helpful for those experiencing something resembling low desire or for couples with mismatched libidos. Sometimes we have to "get in the mood" to *get in the mood*. Relying solely on biological impulses like horniness is like waiting for a bus that just never comes. That eventually takes its toll and can leave us feeling defective.

But it's not *us* that is defective; rather, the beliefs we have about how sex *should* be are reductive. They are limited and based on outdated ideas about human sexuality. We have been square pegs shoving ourselves into round holes. It just doesn't work. We need to update the models. We need to change the way that we understand human sexuality and be more inclusive of a variety of experiences.

5. Men and Women Are Opposites

Moving on from here, the last myth that I want to bust is the idea that there are extreme desire differences based on gender. While traditionally, the philosophy has been that cis men have higher sex drives than cis women, what I am seeing increasingly in my work and in my practice, now backed up by mounting data, is that this is untrue. I'm increasingly meeting cis women in heterosexual relationships whose sexual desires are much, much richer than that of cis men, specifically their cis male partners. And I am also seeing people in LGBTIQ relationships where desires are not well matched—none of which have anything to do with gender.

Sometimes, sex problems can lead to emotional problems in a relationship, especially when a lack of enthusiasm for sex is interpreted as a lack of love or affection. The idea that the default setting for all cis men is that they're going to be horny and aroused and constantly chasing sex, is a really unhelpful, boring, and inaccurate idea. It lends itself to so many misunderstandings based on limited knowledge of sex and gender. For example:

He doesn't want me. Does that mean he doesn't like me?
He's not chasing me, he doesn't want sex.
I have to proposition him for sex all the time and he knocks-me-back.

And for heterosexual cis women, that can be experienced as especially affronting because of the belief that cis men are hard-wired for sex at all times *no matter what*. So to be knocked-back in this way is not only confronting but downright offensive, especially when we collectively expect cis men to operate in this truncated, soulless capacity, simply to fit a stereotype.

Part of understanding what desire means to us is letting go of the ideas we have been led to believe about sex, gender, hormones, and libidos. In some cases, the presence of testosterone increases libido; this is often true for people taking testosterone for gender affirming purposes and occasionally by cis women for so-called low libido—but not permanently and certainly not as a cure for so-called frigidity. There is no hormone, pill, or injection that will make us comfortable with sex if we simply aren't or or desire sex that's unfulfilling. There isn't a pill that will make our lovers more attentive and tuned-in to our needs. The way that cis men and cis women are taught about sex varies greatly, not to mention how non-binary and gender non-conforming people are left out of the equation entirely, all of which likely has a far greater impact on how we experience desire for sex than anything coursing through our veins or between our legs. Traditionally, cis men were taught that sex was not only something they are *entitled* to but also something they should seek at all costs, as part of being "men." This is illustrated in films like *The 40-Year-Old Virgin*, where being a heterosexual cis man, forty and a virgin, is the subject of ridicule. Cis women, on the other hand, have been met with double standards that label them either "slutty" or "frigid," with little space in between. An example of this is demonstrated in the once popular *Fifty Shades of Grey*, where the leading female character, Anastasia Steele, is coerced into a variety of sexual acts. It's OK for the mainstream as long as she maintains a veneer of innocence or purity. Had she been the initiator, do you think this title would have had the financial success it rendered?

These stereotypes are beginning to change and new perspectives are poking through the facade of gender roles and the limitations they have created for connection and quality of life. Slowly, these ideas are being questioned and, in some cases, replaced with more nuanced ideas of what's possible based on feelings and experiences of sex and pleasure rather than obligations to stick to a gendered role. Moving forward, regardless of our age, our sex education is going to have a greater effect on our desire; far more than gender identity, what's between our legs, or even the impact that our hormones have on us.

Creating better sex is about us expanding our knowledge of how desire myths affect us and how gender ideas have informed these myths. The antidote to much of this cultural muddle lies in our ability to be more comfortable discussing sex, our capacity to communicate our thoughts, feelings, and ideas, and how much energy we are prepared to invest in creating a sex life that is as fulfilling as it is meaningful.

In the next chapter we will learn more about the impact of biology on desire, while we explore the relationship of the brain, the mind, thinking, and embodiment to our interest in sex and, ultimately, how this research can help us build our unique erotic templates.

CHAPTER 5

~

Different Kinds of Desire

Sexual creativity stems from living life as if you were making something of it—instead of being made over.

—Susie Bright

In chapter 4, we explored some of the cultural and social ideas and values we associate with desire. We distinguished fact from fiction and laid some foundations to how sex research, while well-intended, set us up almost sixty years ago with some pervasive ideas about human sexuality that we now recognize as wildly incomplete. In this chapter, we'll continue our exploration of sex research through more contemporary lenses, with a focus on biology, and consider how expanding our ideas and experiences of desire can actually help us create more of a "mood" than rely on horniness alone. We will look at the notion of "desire" as a verb, an action, *and* as a state of being, something that we interact with it and how it is contextual—like happiness or fear. We'll continue to examine how useful our *beliefs* about desire and libido are and look even further into what effect their presence has on our ability to connect with our motivations and experiences in sexual encounters and relationships.

The word "desire" has its origins in French dating back to around the twelfth century—meaning, *longing* or *wish*—and rose to prominence alongside its companion "lust" around the same time in Old English.

In modern times, both desire and lust are words that conjure visceral responses within our psyches and bodies—some affirmative, some less so—as the pressure to be *desired* or *desiring* seems stronger than ever (just look at music videos and fashion advertising to see how it manifests) with little reference or context for it. Sexy images appear rather innocuously everywhere to sell everything from alcohol to zucchinis, unconnected to the products but effective in getting our attention. It's not that erotic imagery is a bad thing by any means, it's not. It's simply that, despite it being the undisputed muse of pop culture, the majority of us still struggle to talk about sex in useful or meaningful ways.

Increasingly, we are much better at watching sex than we are at doing or even communicating about it; we have not yet caught up with how to manage ourselves, our feelings, or our behavior in its presence. In fact, it's the unrealistic relationship we have created with desire itself that has borne so much suffering and misunderstanding. Allow me to explain.

Many long-term couples I see will tell me:

"You know, I love my partner but we don't have sex anymore."
"We haven't had sex for three or four years."
"We haven't had sex for two months."
"We don't have sex often enough."
"Sex between us has really dropped off."

Frequency is almost always the sole determiner in measuring how satisfactory their sex lives are. And as we learned in chapter 4, the frequency of sex tells us nothing about its quality.

When I inquire further, they tell me:

"I want sex to be spontaneous. I want it to be like it was in the beginning."

Because, most often, when we think of desire we think of *spontaneity* and *passion*. And in many ways, that there is the problem in and of itself. The sex that people long for is the sex they (sometimes) experience at the beginning of a relationship. The heat, the passion, the carefreeness of it all—combined most effectively with not knowing or even caring if you are going to, in fact, be able to "have it all." The urgency of desire is focused on the rush of possibilities, which offers an escape from our daily lives. It's a brand-new context for us and thus it's exciting by default. It's the antidote to the strains of domestic life, illness, financial burden, or monotony of routine. In some ways it explains why erotic imagery is so popular in advertising and pop culture. It allows us to escape from the day-to-day.

Spontaneous Desire

Even the phrase alone conjures images of youth, tropical vacations, cocktails by the beach, and random acts of lust in the back seat. The longing many of us have for spontaneous sex is not so much the idea that we're just walking down the street and then BAM, there we are having sex on gritty, grubby terrain. Rather, the abandon we long for is richer; speaking more to an experience of recklessness than to sex itself. It's what spontaneity *represents* that lures us in. It gives us a break from the routine of our daily lives. While youth is synonymous with passion, freedom, and spontaneity, no one over twenty-five would be inclined to take sex advice from a teenager, yet we successfully convince ourselves that hot sex must be like it's portrayed in teen romances—spontaneous and carefree—in order to be fulfilling.

Spontaneous sex offers the prospect of freedom. For many, spontaneous sex is actually completely impractical, but an intoxicating idea. It's the elixir of abandon that eliminates admitting we feel awkward about our relationship to sex and the conflicting emotions it brings us. It's the adventurous thrill of being alive. It's having no more fucks to give. It's the bliss of ignorance. It's being free of inhibitions, burdens, and the discomfort that comes from having sex within an emotional transaction that matters—like a long-term relationship. Yet, despite the hype, many in long-term relationships describe spontaneity in sex as being a major problem. They're not living the dream and they fear the ship is sinking. It appears that nothing is a greater anti-aphrodisiac than the *pressure* to be spontaneous in front of someone whose opinion really matters to us.

Much of what we associate with *spontaneous sex* is not the unexpectedness of it, but rather the passion and enthusiasm of it. The fantasy of getting swept up in the moment is attractive. It offers a balm to soothe any strain we feel broaching the topic with partners; because in spontaneous sex—it just magically happens. We're not responsible, we're not weighed down, and we're not anxiously worrying about who's coming (literally) or what kind of performance we are putting on. We are free of the burdens and tension that arise from facing the realities of making sex a priority. We are the desired and the desiring. And there's no room for confusion. No wonder it's so damn attractive.

However, this is not necessarily the norm. It's not *abnormal* either, nor is it bad, but it tends to be the default many speak of when asked to reflect on desire. While for some a highly-charged libido is something that they can access any time the wind picks up, and on the surface may *look* spontaneous, there is still a *context* in which this happens that allows the flame to ignite. Just like happiness and fear—these feelings generally don't arise out of nowhere. They are a response to something. A thought, a word, a glance, a fragrance, a sensation, a series of text messages are all contexts in which spontaneous desire enflames, but the preparation that goes into them, sometimes even weeks or months earlier, contributes to the feeling of engulfing spontaneous desire.

Responsive Desire

In contrast to the notion of spontaneous desire is *responsive desire*. Just like the moon's effect on the ocean, responsive desire is as it sounds, a *response* to some kind of stimulation or arousal, or having certain emotional, physiological, or environmental "conditions" met.

Looking back at Basson's "Human Sexual Response Cycle" in chapter 4, responsive desire follows the notion that if *arousal, interest,* or *motivation of any kind* is present (arousal being engorgement, lubrication, erection, flushed skin, etc.—any of the physiological aspects), then desire may come more freely after that. In other words, getting to the place of *wanting* to "get it on" can come after we have actually started being physical or it may arise in response to something emotional or otherwise contextual—just like happiness or fear.

This sits very much in contrast to the way we have been taught to understand sex and desire. Like the old model from Masters and Johnson (chapter 4), most pop psychology articles about desire and libido insist that they are

a) inherent within all of us;
b) essential to good sex; and
c) must be present for sex to be good.

This is effectively a lie.

If the conditions for "good sex" are met first, the desire for it *may* come along afterward. These conditions could be anything from being freshly showered and knowing there are clean sheets on the bed, feeling acknowledged and validated, not menstruating, making sure the kids are asleep, no threat of interruption, or engaging the right kind of stimulation to activate the pleasure and arousal receptors in our brains and bodies. Traditionally, this form of desire has been associated with women but the truth is that "responsive" desire influences people of all genders—inconsistently at different times in their lives based on a variety of factors including hormonal changes, emotional turbulence, relational factors, environmental factors, stress, and, also, pleasure. While desire was originally conceptualized in early sex research as a *trait*, either high or low (something that was inherent to the person themselves and unchanging, like their height or eye color), responsive desire sees libido as a *state*; something that ebbs and flows depending on the context in which it's happening. Much like the way we engage with the rest of our lives—it's a response to something in our mind, body, and environment. We may be aware that it's temporary—even if, at the time, it feels all encompassing, as if it's all or nothing. While it's true some people are more libidinous than others, just as some are more easily excitable, curious, or introverted, there is strong evidence that affirms that even elements of *trait* desire are still affected by variables such as life events (e.g., pregnancy), relationship or partner factors, and stress. Further still is the theory that when we allow ourselves to explore our desire without shame or repression, this can help shape trait desire over time.[1] In other words, the more we practice "getting in the mood," the more likely it is we will.

Time for Reflection

Take a moment to consider if your desire type is responsive or spontaneous. And you could be a little of both depending, of course, on the *context*.

If you feel horny and desiring of sex at seemingly random points throughout the day or recognize horniness before your body has a chance to get on board, or you're the one who often initiates sex or wants it more often, you may be more inclined toward a spontaneous desire style.

If you rarely think about sex or it doesn't sound like a good idea but once you're doing it you think, *oh, this is great! I should do this more often,* or you are often waiting for the right set of conditions for the mood to strike, it's likely you're more inclined to a responsive desire style.

Knowing this information about your desire type, how could you have more understanding of yourself? Of your partner? What could you share about yourself with your current (or prospective) partner? What is easier to understand now that you have this framework about desire styles? Write this information in to your notebook, as it informs an important aspect of your erotic template.

The Dual Control Model

The Dual Control Model takes the notion of spontaneous and responsive desire even further. The Dual Control Model was developed, during the 1990s at the Kinsey Institute, by Erick Janssen and John Bancroft and differs from other models in that it describes not so much *what* happens before, during, and after sex, but offers a theory on *how* it happens. In short, it references two systems of sexual stimulation: acceleration and inhibition; an accelerator and a brake. The acceleration system SES (sexual excitation system) and the SIS (sexual inhibition system) functions like the brakes.

The core principle of the Dual Control Model is that sexual arousal and response result from a balance between inhibitory and excitatory mechanisms of the central nervous system and the brain.[2] Its strength is informed by evidence of how not only the brain but also the body respond to sexually stimulating input.[3] But here's what's interesting, the focus is not just on that which stimulates but also on what inhibits. Previous models had explored only that which stimulates, but this model looks in-depth at what inhibits us sexually, at a neurological level. The theory goes that the brain and spinal cord encompass a complex and individual combination of brake and accelerator pairings within us. To that end, the accelerator and brake are linked to the autonomic nervous system, which activates both our excitement and reluctance for sex.[4] The sympathetic and parasympathetic nervous systems within the autonomic system are responsible for sending signals between the brain and body to *get excited* or *watch out*—but in ways that do not register at a conscious or even logical level. In other words, we may be both physically excited / aroused and on guard at the same time but for different, or even opposing, reasons. This is often believed to be one of the core issues to address when we experience a problem with our sexual desire or interest.

The SES processes information about sex in your immediate environment and sends information to your body, including your genitals, that sex is coming, so "get ready and turn on." The SES operates at a level that is beyond our cognitive awareness; in other words, it's operating without us even knowing or noticing it. Much like our body's ability to digest food, it just happens without us having to pay much attention to it. We pay attention to what we like to eat, but the rest happens automatically. You generally don't know what's happening until all of a sudden you're feeling horny or turned on, ala *spontaneous desire*.

The SIS is the brakes system. Inhibition is not connected in any way to introversion or shyness but is, rather, a brain mechanism and nervous system response that the body interprets as "turn off." From the research, it is understood there are two components to the brakes. One part is the opposite of the accelerator, assessing the environment for potential threats that will "inhibit" sexual activity. Pregnancy, worry about STIs, or a lack of physical safety are common examples of reasons not to "get it on." These are external situations that cause us to be disengaged in the moment. It's the process that hits the brake when, in the middle of sex, someone unexpected walks in and disrupts proceedings. It's also the system that prevents us from engaging in sexually inappropriate behavior, like in line at the supermarket or during a meeting with your boss. It's not all bad; in many ways it's there to protect us. The other part operates more like a hand brake, as described by sex educator and author Emily Nagoski: "If you try to drive with the handbrake on, you might be able to get where you want to go, but it'll take longer and use a lot more gas."[5] While the first brake is about external consequences, the hand brake is about internal feelings and ruminations such as worries about not having an orgasm, taking too long, not being hard, feeling unattractive, not doing it right, or having too high an expectation in relation to a partner or encounter. The two brake systems appear to operate similarly, even though they process different kinds of information that prevent us having a good time during sex. It's not all doom and gloom, however, as the evidence confirms that while such processes are real and extremely powerful, they appear to be somewhat changeable.[6] This is good news for those of us whose brakes or accelerators are a source of shame and difficulty in our sex lives. A sensitive brake is the strongest predictor of sexual problems in all genders, while some of us are more affected by internal criticism and distractions, others are more affected by external inhibitors.

It's helpful that we recognize these systems within us as a way of understanding our sexual selves better. When we experience an imbalance sexually, this model provides a way of understanding that the cause is due to a discord between the brakes and the accelerator. While each person's brake and accelerator system are unique, there are many commonalities based on gender and sexual experience.[7]

Sexual Desire versus Sexual Drive

The phrase "sex drive" is a common and colloquial turn of phrase. It implies a biological imperative—a burning need that must be sated. It implies something that's uncontrollable and a fundamental requirement for retaining life and balance. But if sex were a drive, *everyone* would experience it in ways that are recognizable—like hunger or thirst or sleep. Recognizable drives are such that people and animals can identify with, no matter their cultural background or gender. Without these things we would die, plain and simple.

Sex, however, is different. Your sexual desire, in contrast, is not a drive. It's at once both a choice at some level, and a response to the conditions that surround your sexual expression, the conditions that pique your interest, the stimulation required to sustain it and the circumstances and mechanisms that distract you from it. You will not die from too much sex or a lack of sex (no matter how much you think you might). But you could certainly have an affected mood as a result of a lack of sex, especially if you experience a lot of spontaneous desire. Your emotional motivation to continue to invest in the chase, the partnership, or even in yourself and your well-being can most definitely be affected, which in turn may affect the equilibrium in your life.

Desire is so much more than simply a physiological drive that is designed to satiate the body to prevent death. If nothing else I urge you to recognize that it's a state of mind,[8] a relationship to life, a sequence of cultural, social, and gendered privileges as well as an experience of embodiment. Desire is an attitude. Desire is a motivation. Desire is a form of willingness. While monthly cycles and the presence or absence of hormones like estrogen and testosterone have been shown to have an effect on the physiological incentives to engage in sex practices, the results are inconclusive.[9] While some cis women taking hormonal contraceptives report dramatic changes to their desire level, others do not at all. The same applies to cis women taking testosterone for low libido, the results are inconclusive as a sole mechanism to increase desire. Similarly, cis men experiencing low desire may or may not display low testosterone levels. Collectively, this inconsistency in framing libido solely as hormonally driven doesn't allow at all for the contextual experiences in which desire arises, nor the ways in which it has meaning as we explored in chapter 3. While some of us are profoundly affected by hormones others are not. This means that things like aging and menopause alone, without context, while relevant, may have less impact on our libidos than originally believed. There is greater evidence affirming that our ability to enjoy sex remains robust right up until we hit the grave, provided we make it a priority, which we'll explore in greater detail in chapter 7. Hormonal interventions help *some* peop' ~ *some* of the time but are not a sure-fire cause of desire in and of th'

Beyond that, the definitions of "help" when unpacl desire are broad and inconsistent. Helping people to · simply do not want is like helping children to eat veget If they don't want them, they simply do not want th' may be good for them. However, the difference is, many people with so-called low libido or partners in mismatched libido relationships often want for it to be different. They want to want it. They want to connect sexually. They want to experience a different relationship with sex and this is possible—provided they are willing to address unhelpful expectations of "normal" sex, outdated understandings of desire and gender, and embrace new possibilities of sex that this book is dedicated to exploring. In short, we have been tricked by bad definitions of sex and even worse media by articles emphasizing sexual "normality" that are woefully out of touch with what motivates us to be subjectively interested in sex. There is simply a much broader range of motivators for sex than just desire alone.

The Brain on Desire

As research continues regarding the brain's relationship to sex, so do the evolving theories of how our brains interact with our sexual preferences and desires. In an interview with former neuroscientist and professor of psychology Jim Pfaus, I learned that, despite our knowledge of brain science and the evidence we have to date of its function, its capacity to change and morph in response to its environment is potentially greater than our research can keep up with. "Brains get used to bad sex," he tells me. "The brain acclimates to whatever becomes normal—where sex becomes unimportant, it's easily remedied by changing the situations to change the brain." This is great news for those with low desire and seems simple enough, so let's see how it works.

The idea that we are our brains, and solely our brains, is a misnomer. We are not our brains any more than we are our eyes or our asses. What happens *in* our brains affects how we experience our bodies, our emotions, and our minds, but the complex relationship between these entities is only beginning to be understood. You are an embodied being and your brain enables your body to do its thing. But your mind is the conscious interpretation of the brain's final output.

Professor of Philosophy at the University of British Columbia and mindfulness teacher Evan Thompson, PhD, describes the function of embodiment like that of a flying bird. A bird needs wings to fly, but the bird's flight isn't inside its wings, it's a relationship between the whole animal and its environment. Flying is an embodied action. Similarly, you need a brain to think or perceive, but your thinking and perceiving isn't actually inside your brain, it's a relationship between you and your environment. Cognition is a kind of embodied action, but it's not in your brain. It's in your *mind*, which includes your brain but also includes other people, practices, beliefs, stories, and values that inform your interactions.

In a sexual context, your mind exists everywhere including your body, which includes your genitals. And your mind includes your way of being in relation to others—your lovers, your partners, your friends, and your broader community. You may not have control over the emergence of your emotions or even your thoughts about sex, but you have control over how you respond to them and how you behave. This is where my interest as a sex therapist lies and where sex therapy becomes extremely useful.

But for the purpose of addressing what is known about the brain, sex, and desire, it is well documented that the old part of the brain that governs sex is the mesolimbic part, often referred to as the "lizard brain." This part of the brain is made up of a variety of parts that work in unison and are centrally located (believed to be the oldest parts of our brains from an evolutionary perspective) and shared with our mammalian and even non-mammalian counterparts. These parts include from the mid-brain periaqueductal gray, through to the medial regions of the diencephalon (both hypothalamus and thalamus) to basal forebrain nuclei; ranging from the bed-nucleus of the stria terminalis, preoptic area, septum, and basal ganglia (e.g., the nucleus accumbens), up toward the amygdala, insula, and several medial frontal lobe structures (including the anterior cingulate cortex, orbitofrontal cortex, and medial prefrontal cortex).[10] It's not essential to laypeople that we know this; however, it is interesting for those inclined.

Together, these parts of the brain govern all of our emotional systems including our seven basic emotional systems: seeking, fear, rage, lust, care, panic, and playfulness.[11] Because all our emotions are centrally located here, from a brain science perspective, it's not surprising then that we feel or experience multiple, sometimes conflicting emotions and sensations at once. In pop psychology articles, this area is often referred to as the "pleasure center" or the "reward systems" area of the brain, however it's more accurate to conceptualize it as a "well-being system,"[12] as these parts work together in an attempt to regulate our well-being. Where the *pleasure* components are addressed is in their functions regarding liking, anticipating, wanting, learning, or expecting—aspects of this old lizard brain function that lights up affirmatively (or not) in response to the presence or even the indication of stimuli—such as sexual activity. The "liking" aspect is the visceral response to some kind of input stimulation. A touch, a kiss, the smell of bacon cooking, or the taste of chocolate can all activate an immediate "liking function" that is more automatic than cognitive. We don't have to think about it. We know if we like something immediately—which is especially obvious with food but, in some cases, less so with sex.

Wanting, however, is different. Wanting in this context can be activated by either innate longings (things we like "just because"—sweets, winning sports games, or being appreciated) or learned incentives— think Pavlov's dog salivating at the sound of the bell. But it's not the bell that he wants, it's the snack that he associates with it. The bell is simply a cue that the good thing is (maybe) coming. It alerts him to pay attention, to be vigilant, even if he doesn't want to be. "Wanting" is often linked with the infamous neurochemical dopamine, which, contrary to popular opinion, is neither addictive nor connected with "pleasure" but rather with incentives and the attention we pay to them. The purpose of an incentive is to tell us we should pay attention or be curious *in case* a reward (pleasure) is coming. Incentive also makes us vigilant—which can work for or against us as we will find out shortly. Regarding pleasure, it's opioids that create pleasurable sensations, not dopamine—but I digress. "Wanting" is determined by what the brain (and your conscious mindful interpretation) has come to regard as familiar or probable based on instinct or a learned response. And although a lack of dopamine can inhibit incentive, there are a host of other brain chemicals, functions, and hormones at play. Combined, they have a powerful impact on determining the things we want, or do not want, and how we respond[13] "because dopamine" is not a robust enough descriptor of how "wanting" works in the brain. Similarly, just because something attractive is presented to us, it doesn't mean we will always want it. This is not a simple equation but seems to have something to do with the context in which it is received. What is desirable in one context, is simply not in another. Ice cream on a hot day may be much more desirable than ice cream on a cold day. The response is visceral, not cognitive. We don't want it and we don't need to think about why. The ice cream is the same—the context determines our response. Sadly though, not wanting sex, unlike not wanting ice cream on a cold day, comes with a slew of social and cultural ramifications. Its value is significantly elevated. People make relationship and life choices based on sex. Less so based on ice cream. So, the stakes here are much higher.

The "wanting" aspect of brain function is not limited to affirmative things but is also linked to dread and aversion—the opposite of "wanting," in the conventional sense. This happens in a variety of ways, most commonly when the context in which the "wanting" happens is changed; the brain learns to associate the feeling of "wanting" with a sensation of anxiety or fear, aversion or boredom—thus producing a recognizable sense of underwhelm or even dread. Consider how many times we've had an experience traveling, singing karaoke, playing sports, or doing some other fun activity that we want to do again and again? But if we did that *exact thing* in that *exact context* over and over—how much fun would it continue to be? From an incentive point of view, it makes sense that we want to repeat the experience—but it is in this exact situation that "we end up in danger of imposing habit on the very thing we love" Pfaus tells me, and thus, in clinging to the same incentive, we also can destroy what it is we long for. In doing so we train our brain to associate the thing we love with repetition. Repetition reduces dopamine production, which reduces incentive, especially when there is no drive associated with it, like with sex. We can cease to want the thing we want! Excitement gets replaced with boredom and the brain acclimates to that. The brain, in this case, is primed for something tedious or unpleasant and expects it—whether it's real or not. The body is then on alert to avoid it or protect itself from it, not move toward and pursue it. Such vigilance, as mentioned earlier, becomes a hindrance rather than a help. The initial learned response of wanting the fun thing is reversed, and the "wanting" becomes a "wanting to get away" from the fun thing, in this case, maybe sex.

Due to the complex nature of this brain activity in conjunction with the interactions of life events, neurochemicals, various nervous systems and hormones, it is possible that we can end up liking things we don't want, or want things we don't like or feel anxious about things we want to like, or be disgusted by things we want to like, and so on. This is especially evidenced in people living with PTSD (post-traumatic stress disorder) where the brain has been stimulated in such a way that unpleasant emotions and responses are produced even if there is no actual threat present.[14] The brain has become conditioned to emit an unpleasant response to stimuli and does so whether there is a genuine danger or not. How our lizard brain responds, and how our cognitive longings or desires actualize, are not always complementary. But the good news is, it is far from a lost cause. When this discord between mind and brain / body becomes most evident in a sexual context, we may experience internal conflict between:

- wanting to want something (wanting sex with your partner—[it's a good idea], but not feeling horny)
- liking something but not wanting it (getting turned on by something you saw in porn but having cognitive aversion to it—*eeew that's gross*—but *I secretly kind of like it*)
- wanting something but not liking it (we forget why sex used to feel good—variety and excitement—not the act itself necessarily—*I used to like sex but it's boring now*)
- not wanting something we used to want (context has changed [kids + sleeplessness + stress + pressure + routine] and the environment no longer stimulates us, e.g., ice cream on a cold day)

And, in addition, we may experience the whole gamut of personal, cultural, religious, and social reasons people feel conflict between their visceral longings for sex and their emotional and cognitive reasons for sex.

Even though brain science regarding sex is in its infancy, it's been well established that brain function regarding our responses to perceived or actual stress are in fact malleable.[15] The feedback loops between the brain's reactions, the body's responses, and the mind's interventions indicate that the autonomic nervous system (which regulates communication between the brain, the body, and the mind) is, over time, able to reroute discombobulating communication pathways between the sympathetic nervous system (associated with fight / flight behaviors) and the parasympathetic nervous system, which helps us relax, be present, and enjoy ourselves. In other words, over time it is possible to change our relationships with our brakes and our accelerators. It's "our attitude that makes the difference" Pfaus assures me.

So at the end of a rather substantial chapter of science, the implications of all this boil down to several factors.

First, desire is far more nuanced than simply wanting or not wanting sex. We know from both brain and nervous system research that above all else, *context* matters, no matter our gender or orientation. In the next chapters we will dive further into what constitutes ideal contexts based on our own individual erotic templates and how to create them. We also discovered in this chapter that sex is not a drive but a relationship to life and to pleasure itself. How we experience desire is dependent on many parts of our lives; and our understanding of hormones and horniness alone are not only grossly oversimplified but woefully inaccurate. We also learned that desire is something that we can cultivate, and while our wiring informs our capacity to experience desire, research confirms that it's not hard-wired. So for those who have once experienced desire and want to want it again, the good news is research suggests it's absolutely doable. The remainder of this book takes the clinical data and theories we have just examined and teaches new applications in a variety of practical ways. Together we'll help you make meaning of your experiences, learn how to talk about what's going on for you and why it matters, and build your erotic template to ultimately help you to stop struggling and start loving.

CHAPTER 6

Looking Forward by Looking Back

Tension is who you think you should be. Relaxation is who you are.

—Chinese Proverb

If you're reading this book in chunks, you may have decided to skip over some of the hefty science content of the last two chapters and this is, of course, fine. From here we dive into how to discover your unique erotic template, including what motivates you to have sex when you do (or used to), why motivation matters, and how the myths we have learned about sex hinder us from really bringing more of ourselves to our sexual encounters and, ultimately, to our relationships.

Why Do You Have Sex?
When I ask my clients this, they often look at me like I've lost my mind.

Why? What? You're the sex therapist. Why don't you know it? You should know the answer to this question.

But then it dawns on them that maybe there is some magic in this question. The reason is twofold. When I ask people why they have sex, they are often able to tell me *how* they have sex, how many times they do it, and sometimes even whether or not they *enjoy* it. But recognizing *why* they have sex takes a bit longer.

This is the single most powerful question in my toolbox as a sex therapist and now yours, as a person who wants to want sex, because the answer to this question helps you expand your knowledge of what motivates you to have sex . . . especially if you find desire a bit tricky. This is why it's a magic question. When you can answer it, you are much more able to understand your motivations and therefore gauge your satisfaction. It gives you insight into what inspires you sexually (or not) and invites you to find ways to make sex happen on those terms! When you know why you're doing something, anything at all, the impetus to do it is generated within you, even if it's inspired by something external—like a conquest, validation, or developing a better relationship. Let me explain.

Imagine if I were to ask you:

Why do you eat the food that you eat?

You would probably be able to give me some very clear reasons without having to think about it too much. They might be about your health, your age, or your financial situation. It could be because you enjoy cooking in a certain style. The possibilities are endless.

Similarly, you might understand that you choose certain clothes because they're comfortable, because you like particular colors, because you like to make a statement, because it reflects your status in the community, or maybe even because you don't much care.

We understand why we do things as straightforward as eating and dressing, so these answers come very quickly and very easily. However, we rarely ask ourselves *why we have sex*.

Could this be because the stigma around food and clothing is negligible in contrast with the stigma around sex? The consequences of our food and clothing choices do have an impact, certainly in religious or highly politicized communities, but these choices aren't stigmatized, they're celebrated. Wearing certain attire or eating from ethical sources communicates our values to the world.

But our relationship with sex is not celebrated—it's disguised and misdirected. No wonder we have such a hard time with it. This is why this question is so fundamental in moving forward in our work in understanding desire and libido on a personal level.

More than Getting Off

For some people, the default response to the question, "Why do you have sex?" might be, "To have an orgasm." This is fine. This is a perfectly good reason. However, if that were the *only* reason that people had sex, we would be satisfied with masturbation alone. And in partnered sex, often we're seeking something else, something *more* than we can experience by ourselves.

One ground breaking 2007 study looked closely at the motivations people describe for having sex.[1] The study found 237 reasons that extended well beyond what most of us associate with simply horniness, including revenge, boredom, money, status, obligation, and celebration. It's no surprise that themes of pleasure and connection were the two most common, or that physical attraction was also popular. This tells us that the idea of sex being simply libido-based is too narrow. Human sexuality is much more expansive than black and white feelings of horny versus not horny. When we limit ourselves *only* to this one narrow motivation, we reduce our opportunities for creating a sex life that's meaningful, the kind of sex life we want.

Having a deeper understanding of *why* we have sex reduces our need to have goal-oriented sex, or certainly decenters it. Goal-oriented sex is sex where the focus is on *outcome* and not on the experience or the process. In other words, the end result rates more highly than whether or not you enjoyed yourself along the way. If your goal is to have an erection or an orgasm, and you don't have it, does that mean that the entire experience of having sex has been wasted? Or does it mean that you could possibly see it in a different way?

How often have you heard that "good sex" means penetration or climaxing? Yet "good" sex is something that many people find difficult to agree upon. If "good" sex is objective, it's something that can be measured and compared, implying we all like the same things.

But we do not. We might be better to talk about "fulfilling sex" or "meaningful sex." That's subjective. Fulfillment takes the pressure off having to perform. It makes it more about enjoyment, like hosting a BBQ or attending a dinner party, rather than submitting a tender or attending a job interview. Knowing *why* you want to do something can help motivate you. It's like waking up on a chilly morning and hearing the rain outside and thinking, "I can't go to the gym today," but getting up and going anyway. You know *why* you're doing it. You want to be fit, stay strong, lose weight, gain weight, get the rush, see that cutie you've been eyeing off, feel healthier, or reduce your back pain. You make yourself go, and once you're there and your blood is pumping, you're sweating, and the endorphins kick in, you think, "I'm glad I made myself do this." Your purpose is embodied and helpful for motivating you. I often wake up too early each morning wishing I'd slept better, *but* I have to get up to take my dog outside. I never, *ever* "feel" like it, especially if I've slept poorly, but I do it because I love him. That's my motivation. And often, once I am out there, I enjoy it too, even though left to my own devices I wouldn't have bothered making the effort if it weren't for his sweet puppy-dog eyes (and the threat of poop on the floor).

Sometimes sexual arousal (the physical engagement) comes before desire (the mental / emotional component—Basson in chapter 4) just like in dog-walking, just like in sex. The trouble with goal-oriented sex is simply that our capacity for satisfaction is limited. Instead, we can expand on this by setting different intentions around our sexual play, and this also offers options for intimacy that do not involve genitals yet still provide for profound connection and pleasure.

So . . . Why *Do* You Have Sex?

Your personal and specific reasons for having sex are fundamentally important. If you don't know *why* you are doing something, it is very difficult to know how much satisfaction you can get from it. Many people engage in sex therapy, determined to answer the questions:

Why don't I want sex?
What's wrong with me?

But struggling for years with the machinations of these questions reduces your capacity for meaningful erotic inquiry. Knowing what's "wrong" with you will likely not help turn you on or help you find out what brings you pleasure. Unless there is an obvious answer that is satisfactory for you, it's much more helpful to reframe the question to ask why you *do* want something, rather than why you *don't*. And in all my years of experience, the answer to, *Why don't I want sex?* never, ever changes anything.

Discovering Your Erotic Template

Case Study: Lonnie
Lonnie is an educated woman in a twenty-five-year marriage. She and her husband love each other without a doubt, but her interest in sex is zero. She came to see me because things had gotten so bad that her husband had flagged ending the marriage due to her lack of enthusiasm about sex.

She knew he wasn't being unreasonable. She was not interested in sex. She didn't hate it either. Just indifferent. She would have sex when he wanted to, more or less, but wondered what on earth was going on when she could go for months without even thinking about sex. She wondered if she was damaged or broken. This was how our relationship started.

Through the course of conversation, she mentioned that she quite enjoyed sex once she got going, but it never occurred to her to initiate. I explained to her that satisfying sex is about context and response and that one of the biggest inhibitors for sex in long-term relationships is boredom and repetition. Her eyes widened. "Do you mean I am bored with my husband?" she asked. "Not at all," I clarified. "What I mean is that it's possible *your body* is bored. Or your brain and nervous system are bored. Or both. That you have become so accustomed to sex with him, in a certain way, in a certain style, in a certain context—which is secure and reassuring on an emotional level but, at a body level, at a visceral level, doesn't get you firing anymore."

When this happens, people understandably feel helpless. This is why they so often seek out therapy to help move through the awkward emotions that come with acknowledging sexual boredom. "But it's not

Time for Reflection

Thinking about sex as a series of feelings, experiences, values, long-ings, and responses means we are so much more nuanced in our sexual responses than just feeling horny or not. Whether you are currently hav-ing sex or not, the part of you that does want to, or wants to want sex again, is invited to attend to this reflection.

Here are some ideas to get you started:

- excitement
- comfort
- as a favor
- to keep the relationship
- boredom
- for money / gifts / food / finan-cial support
- to feel good in your body
- to help partner's mood
- to try something new
- intimacy
- because you're angry
- out of frustration
- for fun
- guilt
- to act out your fantasies
- to experience new parts of yourself
- to relax
- validation
- habit
- for release of tension
- to reinforce your gender identity
- to prove something
- to reassure the other person
- to help calm your nerves / mind
- to stop the other person from pressuring you
- free time
- to get it over with
- to relieve stress
- to have an orgasm
- to feel wanted
- to feel attractive or desired
- distraction from other things
- exercise
- so you can be owed something
- obligation
- pity
- connection
- to feel powerful
- because you don't want the other person to feel rejected
- to learn more about yourself
- to pass the time
- physical pleasure
- to wake up
- for the afterglow
- because it's expected
- confidence
- procrastination
- to feel better about your skills
- to heal wounds from the past
- to get pregnant
- to experiment
- to cheer yourself up
- to feel "normal"
- because you like someone
- to show off your talents / knowledge
- to help you sleep

Complete this sentence with your own ideas and reflections:
  I have sex / want to have sex because . . .

your fault," I reassured her. "You haven't done anything wrong. It's more a question of reflecting on when sex *is* great for you. What makes it great?" She pondered this for a while and then recalled a weekend some time ago where they were out of the house at a campground by the sea. "But it wasn't even nice," she recalled. "I was just in a different headspace. It doesn't make sense though. I don't even like camping."

Understandably she was curious about the link between the camping and desire, much like Pavlov's dog associates treats with the bell. So I explained to her that it's not that she has a "thing" for camping but rather that how she feels away from the house somehow created permission and context for her to take her foot off the brake (like we learned about in chapter 5). "But it doesn't make sense!" she exclaimed. "Of course it doesn't," I explained. "This is all going on *within your body*. It isn't logical. Very little about sex is. Consciously you have no idea this is happening, but your body is communicating with you, through your brain and nervous system—and this is a *really* great thing."

"But it doesn't feel great." She was confused. The conditions her body was responding to, she didn't especially like mentally, but her body was telling a different story.

"I get that, I really do," I empathized. "But what's great is that your body is responding to what *it* likes—without you having to even think about it. It's automatic. Your job is to acknowledge it and pay attention to it. When you understand the conditions you need for pleasure to emerge and pay attention to how your body responds, the more you learn about what gets you in the mood." Let's see how she did it.

What Helps You Get Your Foot off the Brake?

In chapter 5 we looked at the Dual Control Model that sees sexual interest as an accelerator and brake and takes the position that getting excited sexually is less about slamming your foot down on the gas and more about lifting your foot off the brake. This metaphor helps us understand how our nervous systems respond to pleasure: both excitement and relaxation.

What would help you "get your foot off the brake"? Remember getting the brake to ease off is less about sex and more about helping ourselves relax. And the best indicator of what *will* work is what *has* worked in the past.

For Lonnie, she noticed her body was able to relax *away from the house*. It wasn't logical, nor practical, but it was definitely real. In a new environment, where she wasn't responsible for *anything* except herself, she noticed her body could tune into the idea of pleasure a little bit more. She was able to feel interest and curiosity, excitement even, just by being in a new environment where responsibility and history were removed. Of course, she can't go camping every single time they want to have sex, but that singular piece of information was vital to helping Lonnie understand herself, her body, and pleasure a little bit more in her unique context.

Let's take it further.

In his book *Sexual Intelligence: What We Really Want from Sex and How to Get It*, therapist Marty Klein suggests that sexual conditions that help us understand our erotic template reflect three main areas: [2]

1. Yourself
2. The sexual environment (physical, emotional, mental, and spiritual)
3. Your partner

Thinking about times when you have had sex that was satisfying, allow yourself to reflect on *the context* in which it was happening.

- Was it, like Lonnie, away from your usual routine?
- A new environment?
- What helped make it good?
- How did you feel before the sex was happening and what contributed to that feeling?

Try discussing these with your partner (or a friend if you are not in a partnered, sexual relationship). Practice being curious, like a journalist researching a story, rather than judging or trying to make meaning just yet.

The prompts below are just ideas to get you thinking. It's very important to add your own conditions as they come to you, which may take several days or weeks as you begin learning to think about sex differently. It's also vital to write this stuff down. Just allowing the thoughts to roll about in your head is often not enough to help you remember them. The act of writing something down helps you see it, connect with it, and take the time to really focus on it subjectively and objectively. It also allows you to change it if you decide your relationship with it is unhelpful or unrealistic. If you're in a sexual relationship, consider writing your partner's conditions too. The following suggestions reflect the three categories above for your consideration but you can add more if you think of any.

Knowing the conditions you like or need for sex can be clarifying and confidence boosting and is the next step in building and understanding your erotic template.

Your Sexual Conditions

Conditions	You	Your Partner
Comfort What environments are comfortable places for sex? How important is physical comfort during sex?		
Love / Anonymity / Distance How important is feeling close? Does feeling close turn you on? What about sex after an argument? What sensations does "feeling loved" evoke? Is there such a thing as "too close"?		
Closeness / Intimacy What contexts create this feeling in you? How important is it?		
Hygiene Do you like clean sheets, clean bodies, brushed teeth, removed pubic hair? Do you like the heady scent of sweat and natural body musk and hair?		
Privacy / Audience Do you need to know there is no risk of being "caught," or is the thought of getting caught a bit of a turn on?		

Conditions	You	Your Partner
Silence / Noise Does noise distract you? What kind of noise? Could music help with this? What kind of music?		
Practices Which activities (if any) are *essential* for you to enjoy sex?		
Requirements of Partner Do you like them to initiate sex, be dominant or be romantic, pay attention, build the anticipation? How?		

Give examples and be as specific as you can. The more information you have for yourself about yourself (and / or your partner), the easier it will be to start to see patterns of pleasure emerging.

Some common sexual conditions might be:

- situation-specific (e.g., risk of getting caught, being in a hotel room, being by the seaside in a storm, being away from home, being warm, etc.)
- activity-specific (e.g., lots of oral sex, showering together or shaving each other, wearing particular clothing)
- person-specific if you have more than one lover (e.g., you watch porn alone, but not with a partner, or you enjoy light bondage with one partner, but not with a different partner).

CLARA: Making sure no one is going to walk in on me is really important. That makes it hard sometimes because there are kids in the house, but we make a point of getting away every other weekend. Also, there is something about hotel rooms that I really like . . . it just gets me in the mood.

COLIN: It's really annoying but I like for things to be ordered well in the bedroom. If stuff is messy I find it hard to concentrate. I just make sure I keep that part of my life organized.

RAV: A shot of whisky, actually two shots. It just helps me relax.

MONIQUE: Clean. Oh my God. Hygiene is just so important to me. I take a shower every morning and evening and I keep mints by the bed—just in case. I even thought about having mouthwash and a little spittoon by the bed. Is that too much? Anyway, it's just the way it's going to be. I have embraced that now.

JEREMY: Time is the big thing for me. When I was younger I could just "turn it on," so to speak, but these days, it takes a while for my mind to catch up to my body . . . or the other way around, I'm not sure. But I know I am distracted with work, and stress is a problem for me, so quickies no longer suit me. I know that I need time for it to be fulfilling. That doesn't mean I don't have quickies now and again—they are good to keep the momentum up—but I know myself and I know what works for me.

BRAD: I always initiate—not because I want to, it's just the routine we have got into. If I don't initiate, nothing happens, ever. We are working on it. I am making suggestions, telling her about articles I've been reading online that suggest different positions and asking about things she'd like to try. It's not that she's not into it, it's just it's not on her mind. Talking about it and telling her I'd like more input is a bit tiresome, but it's working, so I'll stick to it. I bring it up in the car. It's less threatening when we are not face-to-face. She responds well then.

After going through the table above, consider which conditions stand out as being important to you for sex to be satisfying? Write down your observations in your notebook. This is crucial information for your erotic template.

In chapter 12 we will get up close and personal with what to do with this information once we discover it and begin to learn how to talk about this and share this information with those who need to hear it, but for now we are just taking the time to explore ourselves, without the pressure to dive any further.

Understanding Your Personal Values
From here, let's side-step sex just a little and shift our attention to the things that matter to us most in life. Because satisfaction in sex is so

much more than just having hot sex, it's also understanding why it matters and which personal values we are seeking to be met through sex, relationships, and connection. Our personal values function like guiding principles, north stars that keep us oriented and anchored to what brings us meaning, purpose, joy, and passion. Values inform our personal, moral, and emotional compasses. For example, security, family, finances, honesty, quality time, and independence are values many people hold dear. These values inform people's choices, like whether to get married. Whether to have children. Whether to buy a house. Whether to buy a car. Whether to be monogamous. Whether to be vegan. And so on. Some of these values are negotiable, others are not.

Let's take some time now to explore your personal values before we begin to apply them to further understanding your unique erotic template.

Get to Know Your Values

Consider your top ten personal values. Some popular ones are listed here, but this is not an exhaustive list. As you read over them, notice which ones resonate with you. Circle them in the list below, or add in any that are not there. If there are more than ten that stand out to you, circle them anyway and you can return to reduce the list at a later stage. Try not to have your final list too long, as it will make working with them that much harder. What's most important is you get to thinking and feeling into what matters to you and brings you meaning and purpose.

Acceptance	Attentive	Challenge
Accomplishment	Awareness	Charity
Accountability	Balance	Cleanliness
Accuracy	Boldness	Clear
Achievement	Bravery	Clever
Adaptability	Brilliance	Comfort
Alertness	Calm	Commitment
Altruism	Candor	Common sense
Ambition	Capable	Communication
Amusement	Careful	Community
Assertiveness	Certainty	Compassion

Competence
Concentration
Confidence
Connection
Consciousness
Consistency
Contentment
Contribution
Control
Conviction
Cooperation
Courage
Courtesy
Creation
Creativity
Credibility
Curiosity
Decisive
Decisiveness
Dedication
Dependability
Determination
Development
Devotion
Dignity
Discipline
Discovery
Drive
Effectiveness
Efficiency
Empathy
Empower
Endurance
Energy
Enjoyment
Enthusiasm
Equality

Ethical
Excellence
Experience
Exploration
Expressive
Fairness
Family
Famous
Fearless
Feelings
Femininity
Feminism
Ferocious
Fidelity
Focus
Foresight
Fortitude
Freedom
Friendship
Fun
Gender
Generosity
Genius
Giving
Goodness
Grace
Gratitude
Greatness
Growth
Happiness
Hard work
Harmony
Health
Honesty
Honor
Hope
Humility

Imagination
Improvement
Independence
Individuality
Innovation
Inquisitive
Insightful
Inspiring
Integrity
Intelligence
Intensity
Intersectionality
Intuitive
Irreverent
Joy
Justice
Kindness
Kink
Knowledge
Lawful
Leadership
Learning
Liberty
Logic
Love
Loyalty
Masculinity
Mastery
Maturity
Meaning
Moderation
Monogamy
Motivation
Non-binary
Non-monogamy
Openness
Optimism

Order
Organization
Originality
Passion
Patience
Peace
Performance
Persistence
Playfulness
Pleasure
Poise
Politics (personal)
Polyamory
Potential
Power
Presence
Productivity
Professionalism
Prosperity
Purpose
Quality
Queerness
Realistic
Reason
Recognition
Recreation
Reflective
Respect
Responsibility
Restraint
Results-oriented

Reverence
Rigor
Risk
Satisfaction
Security
Self-reliance
Selfless
Sensitivity
Serenity
Service
Sex
Sexuality
Sex Work
Sharing
Significance
Silence
Simplicity
Sincerity
Skill
Smart
Solitude
Spirit
Spirituality
Spontaneous
Stability
Status
Stewardship
Strength
Structure
Success
Support

Surprise
Sustainability
Talent
Teamwork
Temperance
Thankful
Thorough
Thoughtful
Timeliness
Tolerance
Toughness
Traditional
Tranquility
Transparency
Trust
Trustworthy
Truth
Understanding
Uniqueness
Unity
Valor
Victory
Vigor
Vision
Vitality
Wealth
Welcoming
Winning
Wisdom
Wonder

Next, consider, what it is about these ten chosen values that *matters*? What does having this value make you *do* or *say* to get it? Is it something you aim to meet through relationships? Through community? Or something you embody on your own?

For example, if you value freedom, what in your life gives you the ability to embody that value of freedom? Perhaps it's owning a car or motorbike. Perhaps it's taking regular vacations. Perhaps it's living alone. Or having a separate bedroom from your partner. Or if love is a value you hold dear, what do you do to demonstrate love? Do you buy gifts? Do you say nice things? Do you make time for the other? Do you like hugs and kisses? Is sex part of love for you? Or if humor is a value you hold dear, how do you ensure it is part of your life on a regular basis? What about security? Is it important to you? How important? How do you make sure security is tended to in your life on a daily or weekly basis?

When looking at your top values, remember nothing is fixed unless you need it to be. Consider which values might be flexible for you? And how? Under what conditions? And which ones are fixed, that you would simply *not* compromise on?

Now a word of caution: try not to turn this activity into an opportunity to beat yourself up for not living according to your values 100 percent of the time. Some of us have the range and resources for that more readily and easily than others, and even still it's unlikely we are *always* able to. There is no right or wrong. Remember you are taking an investigative role here, not being a judge. However, it's an opportunity to reflect a little deeper and explore more of what *actually matters to you* in life, in general, and to see how you are living a life that may support passion, joy, and pleasure—if you want it. Again, you don't need to be in alignment with your values 100 percent of the time on every single thing, but it's a useful road map to help you create more room in your life for the things that matter including a robust sex life, should you want it.

FELIX: Security is a big one for me. I really value security and fidelity. I would simply never go with another person no matter how difficult things are for us sexually at home. We agreed to a monogamous relationship and I am not interested in changing that. I value security which means that I have to find a way to talk to my partner about the variety I want in our sex life. It's difficult when we get these messages that loving someone means you are also going to be sexually compatible. In some ways we are and in some ways we are not. My condition for variety is important and so is my value of security, and one we are working through together at the moment. She is fine with the way we have sex now, but

I am not. I love her but the sex is too routine, too boring for me. This is my challenge.

KEVIN: Duty and honor are pretty important to me. If I feel like I'm putting in the effort to work on our sex life, I expect that my partner is too. If it were just me doing it, and he wasn't, I'd feel pissed off. I appreciate he's with me on this, which affirms my value of love.

SASHA: Family is important to me and so is sex, but sometimes I feel selfish if I prioritize sex over time with my kids. I know it's crazy. I am a dedicated parent, but there is a part of me that feels selfish and guilty if I don't want to see my kids so I can make time for my boyfriend.

GRAEME: I like to be in control. Call me old-fashioned, but I like routine. I guess I am not very experimental with things, including sex. I like things the way I like them. My wife gets annoyed with me.

NATALIE: Faith is important to me. I grew up in the Church and I still believe in Jesus today. Even though I'm not super religious anymore, I don't go to church or anything, I still have faith in the Christian path and I seek out modern interpretations of the Bible to help me manage the purity culture hangover that dampens my sexuality. It's always a work in progress. I love my partner and I am trying.

MANDY: Queer community is a big deal for me. I am in a heterosexual relationship and I identify as queer but my partner doesn't identify as anything. I am still working out how his "non-identity" affects mine and how that affects our sex life.

SALV: Trust is a big deal for me. I trust my boyfriend and he trusts me. Trouble is, I don't trust myself though. I can't tell him I have been having sex with other guys. It would destroy the trust between us, even though it's kind of a lie.

CATHERINE: Intelligence is important to me. So is pleasure. Sometimes, though, I get stuck in my head and I forget to have fun. I really have to remind myself to "let go." It's funny how I can value both passion and intellectual rigor at the same time. I find intelligence such a turn on, it's one of my conditions, but it's also a distraction from getting down to it. Sometimes I get more engrossed in talking about sex than doing it.

Looking at the examples above, we see how some people's values are not always so easy to embody, and how some sit in contrast with what they recognize as their erotic "conditions." Being aware of how their values and conditions interact helps them understand more about what's causing difficulties in their sex lives and in experiencing fulfilment. Now, while this may seem distressing and complicated, bear with me. Let's recall what we learned in chapter 3 about Jack Morin's Erotic Equation (Attraction + Obstacles = Excitement). Morin tells us that desire can, in part, be informed and awakened when the things we want (i.e., attraction), perhaps in this case our values, may be met with obstacles, to create excitement.

One example could be if you, of any gender, value feminism and, simultaneously, one of your conditions is that you enjoy the psychological thrill of rough or humiliating sex with people who identify as female. To an observer, it may seem that valuing feminism would mean you couldn't engage in sex with women in submissive or humiliating roles that may explore this territory, whether you're the instigator or the recipient. However, applying Morin's theory, we could arrive at the conclusion that these two seemingly disparate values and conditions could perfectly coexist *if* there was permission in your inner world and with that of your partners' for the two to somehow blend. In other words, if you knew you could play at that level *and* still be valued and validated as a feminist by you and your partner outside of that play, could it make sex in that context more exciting for you? Or could it make desire more accessible? What could be opened up more by being able to merge these seemingly disparate values and conditions?

Remember the brain science we looked at in chapter 5 helps us understand how we can be attracted to something while also finding it cognitively challenging to accept. For example, we like a thing (perhaps something we saw in porn) but *wish we didn't like* that thing, because it challenges our values or beliefs in some way. And somewhere in this heady mix of brain chemistry, erotic philosophy, and good old self-inquiry, we begin to find a blue print that highlights a pathway back to pleasure and desire.

Take a moment now to consider how your values may interact with your erotic conditions. Could they be distracting, like Sasha, and induce guilt? Could they be liberating, supportive, and affirming, like

Kevin? There are an endless range of possibilities. When our erotic conditions are in sync with our personal values, we may find ease, peace, or even excitement or, conversely, we may also be at the mercy of boredom and frustration, like Felix. Alternatively, when we are out of sync with our personal values, we can feel disoriented and sexually frustrated, perhaps like Salv. Do not despair though. This is *not a problem to be solved* but, rather, a quest to be seized.

In the next chapter, we'll look further into what creates and sustains satisfaction within us and consider further opportunities to understand and engage our longings and desires, including how to make peace with them, communicate them to those who matter to us, and how make them happen *if we want to*. Nevertheless, practicing tuning into the machinations and paradoxes of what inspires us is useful when learning more about what enlightens and stimulates our erotic template.

CHAPTER 7

~

The Triangle of Satisfaction

In touch with the erotic, I become less willing to accept the powerlessness, or those other supplied states of being which are not native to me, such as resignation, despair, self-effacement, depression, self-denial.

—Audre Lorde, *Uses of the Erotic: The Erotic as Power*

In the previous chapter, we explored the interplay of our personal values and erotic conditions and started to work with the notion that knowing *why* we want something is a more reliable pathway to wanting it, or getting "in the mood," than knowing why we *don't* want it, or waiting for horniness to swoop down and magically take us away. We considered how the "erotic equation" may apply to us as we discovered how our motivations for sex, coupled with our sexual conditions and personal values, offer us a portal into creating an erotic template and a sex life that's as satisfying as it is meaningful.

In this chapter, we go further into the importance of satisfaction and consider what is *actually* satisfying for us. We'll discover how to begin thinking about sex and desire in ways that bring us closer to *pleasure*, while we step away from the idea that we should want sex that's ultimately unfulfilling, simply because it's sex.

Satisfaction

When we skim articles about sex in mainstream media, there's often a disproportionate focus on problems and one-size-fits-all solutions. What we are doing wrong. What everyone else is doing. How often we should be doing it. And so on. The formula most of these agencies use is the clickbait tactic. They get you hooked into to their story and then provide a cookie cutter formula for solving the alleged problem, like giving the best blow job or an expert guide to first-time anal. While some of the content might be valid and even useful, what these "hacks" do not offer you is the insight that accompanies how satisfying such activities are and on what grounds or in what context. And let me tell you, the difference between so-so anal and amazing anal isn't the positions you try, how hard he is, or how hard you come—it's how satisfying it is for *both of you*.

Research[1] confirms that being good at a technique, having a high frequency of sex, having dozens of partners, or hooking up with the hottest person on Tinder, while fun, pales in significance if the experience or achievement is not embedded with meaning or purpose based on something that satisfies us *personally*. Within this, no amount of blow job prep or positions ad infinitum will ever get us close to the satisfaction we seek if we indeed avoid inquiring about our own satisfaction and what we want at all. Mainstream sex advice tends to focus on solving "problems" generically, but at the end of the day what we are all seeking is satisfaction, a resolution to our discomforts, and approaches that work for us subjectively. I purposely said "approaches" here because there are many ways to access satisfaction. Given the fluid and idiosyncratic nature of sexual satisfaction, and its propensity to change with our moods, personalities, and life experiences, it's helpful to have a variety of approaches at hand to mix things up a little while keeping the process interesting as well as fun.

It also gives us permission to appreciate the aspects of sex that we may not feel are as valid or as important as others. As previously discussed, most of us are taught to have a somewhat narrow view of what sex is—usually, it has to involve some combination of genitals, or erections, or orgasm. And of course it can, it absolutely can. But also it can involve sensations, feelings, or states of consciousness that add an almost "otherworldly" experience, as if they expand our relationship to life itself.

Case Study: Clara and Theorn

When I met Clara and Theorn, a heterosexual cis couple who had been married for fifteen years, they were in a rut. I usually worked with them together, but during a solo session Clara shared with me that she loved Theorn but, in many ways, she felt he no longer contributed to exciting her.

"I love him, I mean, how can you not?" She looked at me with a raised eyebrow as if to say, "You've met him! He's charming, *everyone* loves him!"

I smile and nod in agreement.

"But he wants sex *all the time*, and it's just not fun anymore. It feels . . . well, needy. It's really not a turn on."

Needy sex. So often the higher-desire partner can come across as "needy" whether they mean to or not. The next time I saw them together, Clara brought it up again.

"But Theorn," she said, "you know you act all nice during the week and then it gets to Sunday night and you're like a puppy, sitting there with the puppy-dog eyes, looking at me wanting sex. It's like, *I've been good all week, now where is my reward?*"

"But I'm horny," he said rather matter-of-factly. "Is it wrong to want sex with my wife?" he complained.

I chimed in, "No of course not, but you two *as a couple* have a problem in the timing of your desires. It's not your fault, nor is it hers, but . . . have you ever wondered what it was about sex that you *actually* wanted from it? I mean, looking beyond the simple explanation: Me Horny. Me Fuck. If you *just* wanted to get off, you could sort *yourself* out, you know?"

In his eyes he was doing everything right. He was a modern husband. He did his share of domestic stuff, was a great father, they both earned good money, and they liked each other still. He didn't get what the problem was.

Theorn looked offended, "But . . . I'm married. I want to have sex with *my wife*."

"I get that," I explained. "And she wants sex too, but she doesn't want it *the way* you do. And because she wants it different, sometimes you sulk. That seems like a strong reaction to have to not getting your rocks off. If you really needed *just that*, you *really* could help yourself there."

I knew it was a tricky statement, but they were in a tricky situation.

As it was, their sex life had all but dried up, so what did he have to lose? After all, a little bit of self-inquiry never hurt anyone. And therapy is not for the faint-hearted, and for people wanting to get to the guts of their sex problems, sometimes the challenges are great.

Theorn and Clara were gutsy.

Even still, Theorn had to take that one home to process. It hadn't occurred to him that his longing for sex with his wife could actually be about *more* than getting off. But what? I left him to consider that. The standard man-box trope was destroying their connection and neither of them were satisfied. I didn't expect him to come up with a clear answer, but I hoped he'd give it some thought. Naturally, this was my way of asking him, "Why do you want to have sex?"—the question to beat all questions in the sex therapist tool box.

He returned the next week, looking very pleased with himself and excited about being there.

"Well, I wanted to say first of all, that what you said really shocked me. It freaked me out actually. I just couldn't get my head around it for a few days. But then, I realized, it's actually *not* just sex I want from her."

He could see from the look on my face I was intrigued. Not only had he really engaged with the question I posed, but he'd come up with something that really resonated for him.

"It's excitement!" he declared. "I mean, I want sex, of course I do, but what I really want, is to feel excited. I want to feel excited *with her*. Sex is how we used to do that, but that's changed now. I still find sex exciting with her, but she doesn't. I've realized what I am looking for is excitement. I want to feel that again and that's what's making her feel pressured."

This was a powerful realization for Theorn. By allowing himself to be curious about what he really wanted, by giving himself permission to accept that his satisfaction was so much more than horniness, he was able to open up to a new way of connecting with Clara that reduced his neediness and invited her into her own pleasure a little more. This is obviously a truncated version of events, but the process remains the same. By both of them being willing to explore their feelings and what needed to change to create satisfaction, they were able to talk about

Time for Reflection

Think of an experience, sexual or otherwise, that was especially satisfying for you. Allow yourself to drift back to the experience. See if you can *feel* yourself there again. Notice how *your body* feels. Notice how your body responds to the memory. Notice what sensations come alive for you. Notice what your mind does when your body is engaged in the memory. For some people, such embodiment quietens the mind significantly. Allow yourself to revel in this memory of satisfaction. What made it satisfying? What personal values were met by the experience? If sexual, which conditions were activated within this experience? Allow yourself to really gather as much information about the experience as you can to get a sense of the meaning it gave you that made it satisfying. Write or draw about this in your notebook. What might this add or open up for your erotic template?

sex in the relationship and consider what else they could do to offer Theorn the excitement he longed for while taking the pressure off Clara to be the sole source of that for him.

A Brief Note on Satisfaction versus Perfection
A *satisfying* sex life is not a *perfect* sex life. People who describe *satisfaction* with their sex lives are never describing perfection. Perfection, if even possible, would suggest a static but temporary state that is likely coupled with anxiety as a reaction to some external measure of success. Satisfaction, in contrast, is a compassionate internal process, informed by self-inquiry, subjective evaluation, and increments of change. Satisfaction requires review and mental, physical, and emotional participation, whereas perfection is finite and locks us into a black and white state of relating to our experiences; things are either perfect or imperfect. Satisfaction, by comparison, emphasizes meaning, nuance, and richness of purpose. Perfection demands we overcome complexity with reason and logic; satisfaction invites us to become curious and fluid—to explore what works for us and includes our feelings, sensations, and values—leading to what some might call ecstasy.

The Triangle of Satisfaction

Over my years in this work, I have discussed sexuality and pleasure with thousands of people. In this time, I've identified three primary qualities and three sub-qualities that people who are satisfied with their sex lives hold in high regard and have in common. These three elements inform the model of relational self-inquiry I call the Triangle of Satisfaction.

I was fascinated to discover that in building construction, triangles are understood to be the sturdiest structures of all. They provide a solid foundation upon which to build anything of importance. Being rooted in three solid points provides a sense of stability for erections (no pun intended), which matched my observations of how sexual satisfaction works in the Triangle of Satisfaction Model. Without these three relational elements, erotic satisfaction is somehow elusive and any sexual formation built without being anchored in these grounds, may struggle to adhere to something more meaningful and desirable.

The Triangle of Satisfaction Model looks like figure 7.1:

The Triangle of Satisfaction

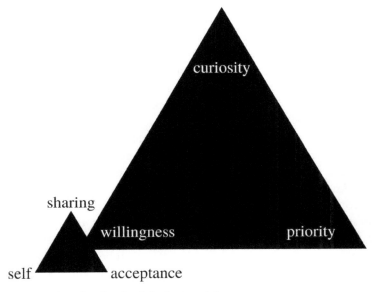

Figure 7.1. The triangle of satisfaction model.

The first anchor point is inviting and valuing *curiosity* about sex.

Sex is many things to many people, including an opportunity to embrace playtime for adults. Think about watching young children playing outside. Not sexual games, just general make-believe games like pirate ships, house, superheroes, or doctors. When very young children play, unfettered and unfiltered by stigma or social taboo, they'll often give their full devotion to the practice. Unless otherwise distracted by fear, shame, or other adult sanctions, they are completely engaged in what they are doing. They are committed to the robustness of their experience, even when it turns sour. They give themselves over fully to the sensations of joy, despair, anguish, and anything else that presents itself moment by moment. They don't filter out pleasure for the awkwardness of it. They are all in, robust, and curious, with little concern for outcomes or consequences. Young children do not stop to ask themselves, *May I do this?* They simply jump in and do it. Instead of seeking permission from some arbitrary inner gatekeeper, they rely on their senses: *How does this feel?* At such a tender age, it's less likely they've started to internalize that intrusive voice that diverts their attention: *Don't do that!* Instead, they remain curious and present to the richness of the experience, whatever it is.

We can benefit from allowing children's engagement with play to remind us what fun *used to* feel like. Leading neuroscientists have proven this with their breakthrough work on the neuroscience of emotions, noting that playfulness actually reroutes our lives toward greater well-being.[2] Studies have conclusively shown that such activity in adults actually rewires our brains back toward pleasure. Many of us have simply forgotten what having fun is about, and in Theorn's case his longing for sex was less about arousal than it was about excitement. For some of us, that enjoyment was taken from us without our consent, which can affect our ability to access pleasure as adults in the short term. And for many, day-to-day responsibilities have taken a toll on our erotic well-being and we've lost connection with the curious playfulness we once, or perhaps never, had the chance to learn. Because adult playfulness is not considered a virtue in many cultures there are few incentives to change. It's helpful to remember we have to put in the effort to get back to that state of permission. Committing to curiosity helps us bypass any internal critique or mental chatter that may otherwise take us out of the moment. For example, an inner monologue during sex of:

This doesn't feel good
Geez I'm bored
I forgot to text Margaret back
I hope my boss approves the proposal
I wonder if Harry got a quote for the patio yet?

(etc.) can all be shifted by applying curiosity:

What could make this better for me?
What am I in the mood for?
What might happen if I put my attention on my nose / chest / face / genitals instead of my thoughts?

When we routinely choose curiosity over habit, a new normal has the chance to emerge. Establishing a new normal can begin with day-to-day practices, not just waiting to do them during sex. When we practice the Triangle of Satisfaction in other parts of our life regularly, it becomes so much easier to apply it during sex too. We can do this by uncovering the answers to:

- How can I (re)connect to childlike inquiry in my daily life?
- What do I need to feel open, alive, and curious?
- What situations / feelings typically shut me down?
- Based on what I have learned so far, how might I approach sex and intimacy in a way that leaves me curious and open, rather than frustrated, resentful, or dissatisfied? For example, What values do I need to bring forward? What conditions could I make sure get met?

Go back to your notebook pages from chapter 2 about recalling an activity you did on two separate occasions that was pleasurable one time and not another. As you look back over that information, what role do you think curiosity played in the time that was pleasurable in contrast with the role it played in the time it was not? If you cannot see how curiosity may have been helpful, do not worry. There will be plenty of time to review at a later stage.

People who experience satisfaction in their sex lives have a sense of curiosity about what they are experiencing during sex, not just phoning it in. They are engaged: thinking, talking, feeling, and playing. Whether partnered or single, this curiosity is one of the core components of remaining in touch with their sexuality. But while sex can be rendered frivolous, curiosity benefits from a sense of worthiness and a recognition of pleasure as valuable, needed, and important.

This brings us to the second anchor point in the triangle of satisfaction: *willingness*. Willingness to try. Willingness to go from one experience to another. Sexually satisfied people are willing to cross the bridge between the old and the new. They are willing to move into areas that are previously unknown to them—even if it feels a little bit intimidating or challenging. Theorn's willingness to explore beyond his initial position of *I want sex with my wife, because it's normal,* allowed him to discover so much more than a quick hand job or ten minutes of intercourse would ever offer him. Sexually satisfied people share a willingness to step outside their daily routine or their regular set of beliefs about how something is, was, or should be. And they combine this with curiosity in some way. They say things like: *You know what? I'm going to give this a go.* They genuinely and wholeheartedly move toward willingness.

This goes back to the important question, *Why do you have sex?* from chapter 6, and the willingness to accept our answers and motivation for what makes sex matter. Your reasons for having sex might not be because you necessarily get physical pleasure from it. You might get emotional pleasure or satisfaction. That is perfectly okay. You might not be a very physically-oriented person. A lot of people aren't. Because our cultural default setting is that you're *expected* to enjoy being touched, this is sometimes where sex can become a problem. I've worked with a lot of people who don't especially enjoy being touched. They don't necessarily hate it, they're just more of a "take-it-or-leave-it" type. Yet they recognize that their reason for having sex is because they want to feel closer to their partner and *that* is what is most important to them.

That is a *great* reason for having sex. All of the reasons that you have sex are great reasons for having sex.

This is why willingness to accept what you find is fundamentally important rather than that self-talk that says:

That's not a good reason for having sex. I shouldn't be feeling like this. I should be wanting sex for the same reasons that my partner wants sex. They are good reasons. My reasons are not good reasons.

Or initially in Theorn's case before he got curious:

I want sex with my wife. There's nothing wrong with that. My reasons are valid reasons for wanting sex. She's the one with the problem. She doesn't want sex (like I do).

That's a very unhelpful yet common internal monologue.

One of the complexities of the willingness anchor point in the Triangle of Satisfaction is that, while internally generated, there is skill and tenderness in sharing and receiving this knowledge.

Willingness is actually made up of three anchor points too. Willingness to embrace what you find about yourself is one anchor. Then there's the willingness to share that knowledge with your partner. Sometimes couples get stuck in expectations of how sex *should* be experienced. And this provides the third anchor of willingness: the willingness to hear and accept information about pleasure and motivations; your own and your partner's. Acceptance needn't mean you have to love it, or even like it, but it does mean there is room to consider it and, if not, a willingness to *consider* making room for it.

It's very common for couples in therapy to say things like:

My motivation for having sex is a bit more emotional than physical. I like feeling close, feeling loved, that's why I do it.

Or remember Rhiannon from chapter 3:

I want sex to make me feel special.

The other partner, who like Theorn might be more physically oriented, might respond initially with:

But I want you to enjoy sex the way that I enjoy sex; or

I want you to have an orgasm (because it makes me feel like a good lover and it validates me); or

I want you to get an erection (because it means I am desirable and it validates me).

Prioritizing willingness to embrace the unexpected, or to accept our different erotic motivations, helps us to deal with obstacles that come up, like a lack of erections or orgasms. (And let's not forget that obstacles are, according to the Erotic Equation [chapter 3], the *essence* of eroticism, so all is not lost). Sometimes it's hard to hear our partners' sexual needs if they are different to ours, especially if what we want is also about feeling better about ourselves.

This is where we can get into problems.

Somehow we got this idea that, as lovers, we have to enjoy sex in the same way or for the same reasons for it to be good. This can be debilitating for many erotic partnerships. In such situations the motivations for sex are less about *mutual* pleasure and more about personal validation whether emotional, physical, or psychological. In chapter 9 we'll take a closer look at how such interactions have become normalized and tend to play out in our sexual liaisons. We forget who the pleasure is supposed to be for and we get lost in a struggle with power and validation, rather than consensual erotic collaboration.

The third anchor point on the Triangle of Satisfaction is: *making sex a priority.* It's really, really easy to forget about sex when we drop into business as usual. We are all terribly distracted by life. Jobs, money, children, pets, responsibilities, family—we've all got a lot going on. Everyone is busy. But amidst the chaos and the busyness, we have to be a beacon of sexuality if we want it to change. And this can be tricky. Really tricky. It's easy to get into a habit of deprioritizing sex. After all, we live in a culture that doesn't reward us for making it a priority, so the effort requires us to be resilient, to challenge the norm and to remember our motivations and reasons for sex.

Making sex a priority is part of the process of developing an erotic template. People who describe a rich level of satisfaction with their sex lives are the same as those who say they pay attention to it. (This is another reminder of how unhelpful the idea that "sex is natural" is.)

We need to put effort in. We need to make it a priority. If we don't put our *attention* on our *intention*, the intention simply won't manifest. It will not come. Not because we are defective, but simply because it's not a priority.

Before we conclude this section, let's consider how the Triangle of Satisfaction might influence our brakes network—the SIS of the Dual Control Model, that we discovered in chapter 5. While the inhibitions we experience in sex may come from a variety of sources—social taboos, nervous system / neurological challenges, historical influences and trauma, gender performances, and so on—getting to know them and how they operate can be helpful. For example, instead of immediately yielding to the brakes and terminating sex, take a moment to consider how *curiosity* might change a dynamic for you. Could you be curious with yourself to consider what needs to change to make things better for you? Would you be able to make asking for it a *priority*? Or what might you be *willing to do*, request, or give to get closer to feeling what you want? Recognize that the brakes are there to slow you down and, at one time, may have been a protection, but they cease to be as helpful when you're ready to move toward curiosity, willingness, or making sex a priority.

What Research Tells Us about Satisfaction

As mentioned in other places in this book, sex is often represented in media and clinical offices as a series of problems to be solved. Clinicians are trained like blood hounds to sniff out problems and trauma, while journalists and writers are now paid per click, leading to sensational headlines rather than useful analysis and critique. While addressing problems and trauma in therapy absolutely matters, and while listicle headlines offer access to information that only decades ago was obscured, our focus remains squarely on what works. What creates pleasure? What creates satisfaction? And what this means for our subjective experience of the erotic in our lives.

Researchers Peggy Kleinplatz and A. Dana Ménard have been researching great sex (not just sex problems) for many years. Their data is especially unique and compelling because unlike research that tells us what's wrong, they offer us a model of what they call "Components of Optimal Sex,"[3] which dovetails especially well with my Triangle of

Satisfaction. Their research has identified eight components of optimal sex, which include:

1. Being completely present in the moment, embodied, focused, absorbed
2. Connection, alignment, being in synch, merger
3. Deep sexual and erotic intimacy
4. Extraordinary communication and deep empathy
5. Being genuine, authentic, transparent
6. Vulnerability and surrender
7. Exploration, interpersonal risk-taking, and fun
8. Transcendence and transformation

These elements are covered in great detail in their book, *Magnificent Sex*, but for our purposes it's helpful to see them distinguished and identified as essential components of sex that operate at individual levels but also at relational levels. This means that changing our relationship to sex, pleasure, satisfaction, and, ultimately, desire is both individual *and* relational. Partners in the "optimal sex" research recognized that, for partnered sex to be satisfying, it took commitment to be real with themselves and with each other. It took them being willing to practice embodiment and presence (more on that coming up in chapter 8). It took remarkable communication and empathy (more on that in chapter 12). It took a commitment to risk-taking, vulnerability, and surrender (more on that in chapters 9 and 10). That is to say, doing the work of creating a sex life that satisfies is a team effort. Sex problems in (consensual, erotic) relationships are never solely one person's fault. They are always at the mercy of a multitude of factors from the personal, social, physical, emotional, spiritual, political, and environmental that merge to create opportunities for connection or disconnection.

Getting Used to New Ways of Thinking about Sex

Most of us haven't been taught to consider sex nearly as richly as we are doing here. And because we haven't been taught, we may be afraid that by taking our foot off the brake we will move too fast. You may fear that, if you reveal too much of yourself, things may go awry. You might worry that you will discover that you are broken or that there's something wrong with you.

Sharing this information can be an intimidating thing to do as you start to take your foot off the brake and move toward a life that is more sexually meaningful. You may feel out of control or unstable. Perhaps concerned that what you discover will be too much. For you? For your partner(s)? For the world? But the fact is, lots of us feel this way about sex because of our collective anxiety about it. Many of us simply rush through sex or ignore it because slowing down to focus on it is simply too anxiety inducing. It's easier to go through the motions with no connection, no reflection, no slowing down to feel it. It's difficult to talk about, so we don't. We keep our foot firmly on the brake because that's safe and familiar.

It's important to remember that when we learn to do anything new, or learn to do an old thing differently, it can feel clunky or difficult. Unlearning is complicated. That is OK. If this were easy, we wouldn't be struggling with sex as a society in the way we do. Making sex a priority, being curious, and being willing are really big deals in a society that actively rewards you for *not* going there. In this way, this work is political.

As author and philosopher, Audre Lorde put it:

> For the erotic is not a question only of what we do; it is a question of how acutely and fully we can feel in the doing. Once we know the extent to which we are capable of feeling that sense of satisfaction and completion, we can then observe which of our various life endeavors bring us closest to that fullness.[4]

- Remember why you want to have sex if indeed you do.
- Remember to explore how to be curious about the kinds of sex that matter to you, and how you want them to make you feel.
- Remember to be willing to engage with what you discover about yourself and you partner(s).
- Remember to make this work a priority, even when it's challenging and you don't feel like it or you're not "in the mood."
- Remember why you decided this was an important thing to do.

Keeping this knowledge in your mind, your heart, and your body is essential for moving past fear or anxiety. Your reasons give you permission to keep going. They give you the capacity to talk about it, to recognize that you are not the one who is broken. *You* are not the only one who has a problem. It comes from the lack of vocabulary around sex and the absence of role models for talking about sex. The fact that sex is still not spoken about in wider society makes us feel ashamed, anxious, and nervous, when sex could actually become part of our permanent repertoire of healthy expression.

I am walking testimony to the fact that this really does get easier. I also had to start at the beginning. I too was brought up in a world that told me it was not OK to like sex, to want sex, and certainly not to talk about it in detail in the way that I do. Taking the initial step—even simply buying this book and reading it—might have been an intimidating or scary decision. But you're here. I'm here. And we are fine. Everything's OK.

In the next chapter we take a look at the role of the body, embodiment, and how the body has ironically become such a taboo in sex and even sex therapy, and explore some ways we can move closer to reclaiming our relationships with our physical selves to create and maintain sex lives that are as nourishing as they are meaningful and satisfying.

CHAPTER 8

The Body Speaks

Sex is emotion in motion.

—Mae West

Before we press on, I invite you to stop for a moment and notice your body. By notice I mean bring your attention to it. Feel it. Its weight. Its texture. Its power. That despite the odds, you are here as a result of thousands of years of evolution, the most advanced form of human life to ever grace the Earth. After the heady learning of sex science in chapters 4 and 5, then the intellectual and reflective self-inquiry of chapters 6 and 7, from here we begin to form a relationship with a vital aspect of erotic intelligence that is often overlooked in traditional sex therapy and indeed most talk-based therapies all together. The wisdom of the body isn't new but, in recent years, has gained a lot of traction in trauma therapy theory as well as its application alongside practices like mindfulness to bring a more holistic understanding of the breadth of the human experience. In this chapter we'll look at how our relationship with our bodies offers us valuable information about sex, pleasure, and satisfaction, and why learning to read your body's language is a crucial step in moving closer to your desire, your passion, and, ultimately, your pleasure. We'll learn some practical tools to get started with using your body as an instrument of erotic knowledge, and we'll unpack how the discomfort we may feel about our sexual inadequacies are not as pathological as we are led to believe.

Having a body is integral to having desire. You could say that the *essence* of desire is embodiment plus action. Desire is a *doing* word, not just an idea. Infused by motivation and incentive *within your body*, this is the organism that transports you around the planet and the vehicle through which you experience the physical world, including the erotic. Desire is personal. Desire gives us purpose and inspires us to action. The desire to consume, the desire to own or have, the desire to *be* (hot, successful, beautiful, rich) influence so many of our day-to-day choices and actions. Owning a home, the latest gadget, having the perfect body, the "hot" partner, reveling in sporting achievements, the correct diet, a new car, or the perfect job are desires many of us are increasingly familiar with. These desires can be fickle or pursued over a lifetime. But our relationship with desire is more complex than simply "wanting" alone. It exists within an environment that encourages or denies it. Depending upon our gender, orientation, age, size, ability, location, resources, race, and the freedoms afforded to us through that, we are at the mercy of how desire influences us and the decisions we make.

In chapter 5, we learned that embodiment is an action that involves more than just the body. We learned how the body is situated within an environment, and like the flying bird, the flight process takes place only within an environment that allows it. Without the interaction between the whole bird and its environment, flight does not happen. When we understand erotic desire as an *embodied action*, we too must recognize that to embody erotic desire, we must interact with the environment that contains it. But when the environment we live neither inspires nor encourages desire in an erotic context, we internalize the taboo in order to make sense of it. In other words, we adapt by becoming disembodied. It's easier to disconnect than recalibrate. We believe we are flawed and we *become* the problem, rather than scrutinizing the systems and beliefs that encouraged it. Disembodiment manifests with stealth. We know we are in its grip when we feel shame or disconnection from our bodies or about our desires. Age, physicality, ability, relationship, and status all affect our access to pleasure. Socially speaking, those in partnerships are considered more deserving of sex and are granted more permission to access erotic pleasure than those who access it via masturbation or paid escort services. Our social merging of love and sex means that sex for some is harder to come by when they do not have access to love. We have collectively made room for sex in the context of a loving relationship, but are still challenged by its presence outside of this. For most of us, pleasure is believed to be something we *earn* rather than something we have a right to. Those more deserving—the slim, young, able-bodied, and so on—are closer to the front of the line than those whose sexuality or body shape sits outside the mainstream view of sexual freedom or desirability. These ideas can have an effect on how we experience desire if we feel that we are unworthy of sex and pleasure.

When experienced in context, desire becomes much more complex than simply being horny or not. How we experience our bodies viscerally and environmentally, combined with our ability to even recognize and accept our bodies' desires is one thing, then how they are situated within our environment is a whole other thing that none of us are exempt from. When the environment we inhabit is not conducive to the emergence of erotic desire, it is increasingly difficult, but not impossible, to connect with this part of ourselves.

When women are forced to continuously deny themselves food or pleasure to prove their femininity and attractiveness (e.g., if you express your desires you're a" slut," you're "too much," or simply "fat") when men are required to deny their feelings and emotions to fulfill the same ludicrous gender stereotypes (e.g., real men want sex, not intimacy or affection), and when non-binary and gender diverse people are robbed of sexuality all together because their existence is just too challenging for the mainstream to comprehend, let alone love, we become trapped in a system that denies the most visceral parts of ourselves at the expense of being accepted and accepting of ourselves. Women become conditioned from an early age that *being desired* is desirable. The nature of subjective erotic desire is foreign to many women. From a young age, girls are rewarded for denying their desires and eroticism to prove their value and worthiness (as wives) later in life. It's no surprise to me that when I ask women what they want sexually, many of them simply respond with: "I don't know." Erotic self-inquiry has never been afforded to them. On the other hand, the versions of desire men are encouraged to pursue are narrow and marked by goals pertaining to achievement and conquest rather than embodied connection. They may know what they are *supposed* to want, but things come tumbling down when they experience a discrepancy between their actual desires and social expectations. When asking men how they *feel*, as opposed to what they *think*, about sex, they will often respond like women: "I don't know." That knowledge has been obscured from the minute they learned that being a "man" meant disconnecting from themselves. Similarly true of gender non-conforming people, as explained by Lucie Fielding in her book *Trans Sex* when she asks, "What if, indeed, the alleviation of gender dysphoria didn't imply sexual losses, but rather the opening onto new possibilities for embodied ecstasy, facilitated by gender euphoria?"[1]

Disembodiment is the physical response to a social agreement that the body is unsafe and sex is shameful or dangerous. Expressions of pure pleasure are, by and large, confronting to those unaccustomed to them. Such expressions are considered shameful and are cast outward, away from ourselves and our communities. This is especially evident when we consider how sex workers are depicted in most cultures, the embodiment of shame that is not revered but reviled the world over. To allow connection with this part of ourselves is terrifying for many. As individuals, there is no incentive to challenge this until the space between our inner erotic and outer physical worlds become intolerable. This is an internal process not visible to the eye, which is also what makes it so treacherous. Subtle reminders of not being desirable or desired, of not being good or worthy enough, of not being eligible to be the desirer because of some shortcoming or simply the absence of erotic privilege to freely choose what you desire because your body doesn't meet an ideal standard of beauty, age, conformity, or function, eventually build a protective barrier making us numb to our inner world. We operate on auto-pilot, and personalized erotic wisdom becomes harder to access. Much like the brakes mechanism, this process begins to shut our eroticism down.

For those with "conventional" bodies, the discomfort of disembodiment may not be acute but rather a state of normality that remains undiagnosed until a catalyst for change, such as a breakdown in relationship or problems with sexual performance, emerges. High functioning, well-respected, socially agile people are no less susceptible to erotic disembodiment; because, this process happens inwardly. The external appearance doesn't reflect the internal experience. For people whose difference is externally visible—people with disabilities, fat people, trans and non-binary people, older people—or those whose bodies feel like a war zone due to abuse and rape or where pleasure has not existed for a very long time, may have learned to tune out of the body for protection. It's safer to disengage.

Before we diagnose ourselves or our partners with "low libido," let's consider all this prior to such hasty statements. Let's consider just how likely *spontaneous desire* is to manifest under these conditions and the extent to which "spontaneity" is a prerequisite for great sex. One of the greatest paradoxes of the human condition is that of our capacity for thought and meaning to the disadvantage of the body through which we experience our lives. Throughout history, the body has been downplayed and undervalued in its ability to produce or hold wisdom and knowledge, as distinct from divine wisdom, or, more recently, logic and science. Previously, guiding principles of conduct and morality were embedded in religious scriptures. In the late nineenth century, science became the leading authority able to determine what a body was and was not capable of.[2] In other words, the body has always belonged either to God or science. There has never been a time in Western history that the body truly belonged to the person who inhabits it.

The Origins of Disembodiment

We are not born into the world separated from our knowledge of pleasure and our body, nor are we born with blockages in our ability to read our body's language and interpret messages of embodiment. We are born whole and integrated, but over time this knowledge is systematically undone each time we experience an individual visceral response that challenges moral conventions. In short, this knowledge is undone in micro-judgments, over and over, once we cease being solely the apple of our parents' eye, (if indeed we ever were) and become a member of society.

For instance, in order to be loved and accepted we learn that chewing with our mouths closed conveys refinement and that sitting with legs apart is acceptable for boys but not for girls, whether it's comfortable or not. We learn that genitals are dirty and anuses are even worse. Girls learn that painful sex is "normal" with no incentive to discover what creates pleasure. Boys learn that sex for girls is painful with no incentive to question it. We are reminded that farting is unacceptable and being fat is disgusting and the result of laziness or a lack of self-control. We learn from a young age that masturbation is unacceptable in public and, in some cases, unacceptable at all times. To transgress any of these is to risk social exclusion and, in doing so, we learn to cut off from our sensations and embodied desires.

This is not just a Western phenomenon. All cultures develop rules of social conduct in order to keep communities organized. Some are useful, others are not. While rules vary from culture to culture, what they all have in common is reflecting a community's values. They describe what a society believes *should* be most important, rather than

Time for Reflection

In chapter 6 we looked at our personal values and how they inform our lives. From here, take some time to reflect on some of the messages and values you have absorbed from your culture about sex, gender, bodies, desire, erotic privilege, who deserves pleasure, who does not, how sex should be, and for whom. Some of these ideas I have introduced in this chapter, and there are likely some that are unique to your culture, community, and context. This might be an exercise you practice over several days or weeks. It can be overwhelming to digest just how much we have absorbed about sex and the body through our cultural context and just how normal it's become to default to shame and stigma when discussing pleasure and desire. Write down some of your reflections in your notebook. Notice how your body feels when you connect to some of these realizations. It's OK to feel many conflicting feelings at once about this, especially if you grew up in a religious environment, in which case this may be extra challenging. This is not about right versus wrong. It's about unpacking what you have inherited through no fault of your own, while giving you a chance to explore how these values may have influenced your beliefs about sex, pleasure, and desire.

anything necessarily factual or evidence-based. Consequently, social rules pay very little homage to embodied wisdom and even less to Eros, because at no time in recorded human history has this knowledge been revered—until now.

The Body as a Vehicle of Desire and Knowledge

Ask any bodyworker and they will tell you infinite stories of how different massage and body work techniques produce a variety of emotional responses in their clients. Responses that transcend remedial pain relief to involuntary release of stored emotion and somatic history. Acupuncturists describe floods of tears. Rolfers witness coughing fits. Practitioners of Alexander Technique facilitate ease with blocked communication. Anecdotally, the lists grow each year. This increases significantly when the attention shifts to the pelvis, a phenomenon also recorded by Dr. van der Kolk's trauma team at the Trauma Center in Massachusetts.[3] What we know now is that information that orients us toward well-being is stored within the body and in order to access its wisdom, we must consult it directly. There is an increasing body of evidence arising from the world of psychiatry and neuroscience that describes in detail how the relationship between the body and well-being is mirrored within the brain. The understanding is that our well-being is bidirectional. That is to say, information about our well-being travels from the brain to the body, but it also travels from the body back to the brain.[4] Knowledge is not just one way. Our capacity for reorienting toward the body, desire, and, ultimately, pleasure is more multifaceted than simply mind over matter. We can actually change our brains by changing our habits. This echoes what the science tells us as described in chapter 5. Our attitude *really* is everything, and our attitude is so much more than just our thoughts. It's also our bodies. Our environments. Our values. Our beliefs. Our spirituality. Our identities. Our privileges. And, as you're discovering, our sex education.

The *rewire your brain* argument has been used with vigor over the past ten years or so by extremist anti-porn crusaders to remind us how such online activity affects our brains. While online activity *does* affect our brains, what is also true is that *anything and everything* we do rewires our brains. The anti-porn brigade is not telling the whole story. Social media rewires your brain. Eating potato chips rewires your brain.

Reading the Bible rewires your brain. Taking time off work rewires your brain. Attending a funeral rewires your brain. A global pandemic rewires your brain. Sitting in front of a computer writing a book is rewiring my brain right now. But the good news is that science is telling us that none of this is permanent. What was wired can be unwired, and it needn't be a top-down process; bottom up works equally as well. This means we can rewire the inhibitions caused by our brakes mechanism by thinking and talking about it; through the mind. We can also change its effects through the way we engage and experience our *bodies* sexually.

In order to develop and expand sexual curiosity, it's helpful to connect and stay with the sensations in our bodies. To experience erotic desire, it helps to explore sensations more fully as a pathway to greater self-understanding. Many psychotherapeutic and therapeutic disciplines such as Gestalt, Emotion-Focused Therapy, Acceptance and Commitment Therapy, Sensorimotor Therapy, Somatic Experiencing, Focusing and Hakomi Method, to name a few, all invite tuning into the body and staying with its responses as a way of making sense of the somatic experiences within. While none of them have any explicit frameworks for addressing sex from a *pleasure* perspective, their foundations are solid and can be applied in our domestic erotic contexts, as I will explain shortly.

The solid evidence of somatic therapies presently focuses on its application to trauma and trauma recovery.[5] Reorienting the body to health and calmness via the body prove viable even in the most severe cases of post-traumatic stress disorder (PTSD). What this implies is that while we know this process works in a trauma recovery context it can also work to reorient us toward pleasure, whether explicit trauma has been present or not.

Growing up as we all have in an environment that enforces disembodiment as a means of social inclusion is, in effect, a traumatic experience. It is not violent in the way many traumas are conventionally imagined, but it's experienced viscerally as a shock to the system. In the same way the bird needs space in order to experience flight, denying the body pleasure offers no way of processing the desires that emerge within us from childhood and beyond. Once the environment no longer supports flight, the bird is captive. In humans, our playful impulses are forced down in a socially prohibitive environment and retired from display. This is how disconnection begins. It explains why so many people struggle with the embodiment of pleasure in their sexual practices. This is especially true of our erotic impulses and impulses of sexuality that defy moral conventions—for example, exploring gender or kink and BDSM, queerness, or homosexuality. In accessing the same principles used in trauma therapy, by tuning into the body for information, we can learn what we need to embody in order to facilitate sensation most useful for developing a language around erotic desire. In working closely with the body and intimacy, trauma is a reason to go slowly, but not a reason to avoid. For others who have simply lost their way, recalibrating the relationship to the body is a liberating process, but one that requires a delicate shift in building capacity from listening with the ears, to capacity managed through acknowledging sensation.

In the past twenty years more has been written on the wisdom of the body, but seldom in an erotic or sexualized context. It seems that bodymind (a term referring to the intelligence of the body) researchers, including the newest recruits of the mindfulness and neuroscience movements are, like the rest of society, deeply uncomfortable with explorations of sex and sexuality. With the exception of Wilhelm Reich, a mid-twentieth-century Austrian psychoanalyst who studied mental health and orgasm, sexuality and erotic pleasure are conspicuously absent from discussions of the bodymind in health and well-being literature. From its initial appearance in scientific texts of the early twentieth century, as decades progressed and sexuality was studied, it was spoken of with diminishing detail regarding its relationship to the experience of embodiment.[6] This stigma plays out in bedrooms across the world and is the primary source of the majority of discomfort people feel about managing their sex lives today. We can discuss sex critically and clinically but are profoundly uncomfortable with its relationship to embodiment and pleasure. This is reinforced by the majority of funding received for sex research, which focus almost exclusively on genital function or reproduction with very little on practices such as oral sex, erotic massage, or anal sex; practices that serve solely for erotic pleasure and increasingly sought in porn search engines and in the boudoirs of sex workers across the planet, due to their immense popularity and curiosity. At the time of writing, Sexological Bodywork is the only established somatic therapeutic intervention that invites clients to experience the body through an erotic lens, via the presence of one-way touch designed to encourage deeper connection and wisdom to the body's innate erotic knowledge and needs.

Facilitating Erotic Awakening

When numbness of the body is a response to sexual self-inquiry or a discussion of what we like is met with "I don't know," it's useful to use that information as a starting point for change. Whether cognitive awareness or sensation are blocked, it can be helpful to remember that such disembodiment is likely to be the result of trauma.[7] This is true for people even without recollection of any *explicit* trauma.

All of us have *embodied experiences* of growing up in communities where expression of sexual pleasure was limited and restricted. We know this because all cultures are in some ways to promote social cohesion, there are some benefits. While not everyone internalizes this to the degree that it's debilitating, almost everyone can recall stories of how they first learned about sex and knew, almost instinctively, that its presence was a source of discomfort.

To manage the discomfort, we learn to disengage. Numbing is effective because we get to tune out. Numbing can be experienced in a physical sense—with no sensation—or in an emotional or cognitive sense, like when people respond with "I don't know" to a question about pleasure, feelings, or desire. Numbing also protects us from getting hurt and being vulnerable. It reduces excitement and anticipation and minimizes the effects of disappointment should they come along. It reduces our need to pay attention, to respond, and, ultimately, to experience ourselves when an anticipated outcome is not actualized, like an orgasm or an erection. When we learn to numb ourselves in order to gain some social advantage, privilege, or, simply, acceptance it's hard to tolerate seeing this embodied in others. And the effect on *our* eroticism and relationship to life is devastating. Just like the bird adjusting to life in a cage, it can survive, but at a cost that only the bird knows—if indeed it dares to feel it. Being numb may be a better option. In order to fit in, we learn to cut off from ourselves and ignore our desires and erotic impulses. This in itself is not a bad skill; the trouble is when it becomes a default rather than something we can turn on and off at will.

Case Study: Lewis
Lewis first started seeing me with his girlfriend when, several years into their relationship, their sex life had started to decline. On paper Lewis had it all. His girlfriend was beautiful, stunning by conventional standards. He had a great job and was respected in his career in law enforcement. But internally, Lewis was extremely uncomfortable with expressing desire. He recognized that if he didn't do anything about it, he would lose her. But his terror was so visceral; it was like he was literally, petrified. His speech was affected. He was slow, uncomfortable with verbal expression and eye contact and this was matched in his body too. The way he moved, the stiffness with which he spoke and walked. Even non-sexual activities indicated a lack of ease in his body. He was simply not comfortable in his skin.

It came as no surprise to me that Lewis experienced frequent problems with early ejaculation and unreliable erections too. Everything in his body was avoiding sex and it was getting out of control. Where his voice was unable to express what he was feeling, his body did very well. What confused him was that it didn't match what he wanted in his heart.

In Lewis's career in law enforcement he had learned to brace himself to threat. This was a useful skill. A survival skill. His sympathetic nervous system protected him very well. His fight or flight mechanism was finely tuned. He was alert to any oncoming danger and able to move out of harm's way in an instant. From an evolutionary perspective, his body was doing what it needed to do.

The trouble was Lewis was also responding like this during sex and intimacy. His body was expressing what it knew how to do when it came to vulnerability: self-preservation. In order for Lewis to experience the kind of pleasure he longed to feel, he had to learn to tolerate vulnerability in bed as well as protect against it at work. While he was set to "on" mode with his body being unable to soften and relax, his body had adjusted in such a way that any invitation for the relaxation of eroticism meant his body jumped in to protect him. His parasympathetic nervous system needed permission to take over at will, to allow him to relax, become aroused, and enjoy pleasure while also practicing the vulnerability of being sensitive and exposed. Whenever his girlfriend tried to initiate sex, he'd withdraw. He'd shut down, find excuses not to follow through. He was protecting himself from the disappointment of his unreliable genitals and avoiding conversation with her about it to avoid the discomfort of being vulnerable.

Over time, she began to feel it was all happening *because* of her. When I met them, she was convinced he no longer loved her. She thought maybe he was having an affair. She too began to internalize his shame. The lack of embodiment in this relationship was spiraling out of control.

For Lewis, the catalyst for change was that he was going to lose his relationship. He knew he couldn't continue as he was, but he knew no other way. This was his incentive. This was his answer to "Why do you have sex?" This was his motivation and his pathway to desire.

Over time, Lewis learned to pay more attention to his body and what was once stiff, cold, and unreliable, became softer and more receptive. But it took time. He and his girlfriend worked long and hard to create erotic scenarios where he was invited to receive touch without having to "perform" by having an erection or an orgasm. Simply being allowed to "receive" touch without having to do anything in response, meant he was able to practice being both vulnerable and safe at the same time. He learned to allow himself the practice of receiving without expectation. This was a brand-new experience for Lewis who had no recollection of being traumatized in sex, yet everything within him responded with fear and discomfort. His physical disembodiment was a response to his environment not allowing him to feel vulnerability, excitement, and desire all at the same time. In Lewis's world, vulnerability meant danger and was to be avoided at all costs. Even though it defied logic, he knew he was safe in bed with his girlfriend, his body responded as if the conditions were not right for him to be embodied. Years of being in an environment not conducive to him spreading his wings meant his body seized up. He internalized the desire to reach out and made it safer to not do it, by not allowing himself to feel his body at all. Using this knowledge to move forward, we were able to craft a series of practices which gave Lewis the opportunity to be embodied in an environment that was conducive to curiosity rather than shame or fear. Sometimes the most direct way back to the body is to use it, and reduce the amount of time spent over-analyzing in the head. Let's see how Lewis did this.

Simple Tuning In Practices

When we allow the body to speak, when we tune in to its language, it tells us what we need. One of the most useful introductory practices to help facilitate tuning in to the body is a simple awareness practice. If you are not aware of what your body needs, it's much harder to enjoy it, respond to it, and, indeed, take care of it or share it fully with another. Learning the practice of tuning in is simple. Staying with it is more challenging. It's a process of tuning in, feeling, and noticing. It's an ever-changing process that invites you to pay attention to dynamics and emotions as they occur. What happens after that, is up to you.

Facilitated by breath, attention, and concentration, the purpose is to practice tuning in to the "felt sense" within our bodies. Philosopher Eugene Gendlin first coined the expression "felt sense" to describe a form of visceral communication between the conscious mind and the physical body.[8] This process is essential when relearning a relationship with desire. When sensation is blocked, so too is desire. In much the same way we tune in to a radio or TV signal, tuning into the body requires getting the feedback just right to receive the signal. It can take practice and time to allow the interference of a chattering mind to minimize enough to start getting accurate information.

Get Centered and Breathe

First, read through this activity before you do it. It's useful to have an idea of the whole activity before attempting it. Find somewhere quiet to be still. Either sit or lie down. Take three deep, full breaths. Imagine a balloon within your belly that expands as you breathe in and contracts as you breathe out. If you are a visual person, see the balloon. If you are a sensory person, feel the balloon. If you are an auditory person hear the balloon expanding and contacting. If you are not sure, try all of the techniques and see which resonate. You may need more than three breaths to do all of this. That is OK. In fact, the more you breathe the more you feel. The balloon is simply a metaphor to remind you that the breath needs to be expansive and not shallow and stuck within the chest. It's bigger and makes everything rise and fall. I call this a "centering" breath technique as it helps you get centered.

Scan

When you're ready, run a "scan" of the body. Imagine a scanner literally scanning the entirety of your body, starting from feet, up to the top of your head. As you run the scanner, allow any "felt senses" to emerge. Just notice them. Anything at all. Do not judge or try to interpret. Simply let them emerge. As they emerge, try to find words to describe them. This is the *beginning* of the process of embodiment.

The kinds of things that we register as "felt senses" include:

- air—cool, warm, direction, rush, moist, feathery, intensity
- itch / irritation—mild, angry, irritating, subtle, small, large area
- temperature—warm, cold, hot, cool, clammy, burning, icy, frozen, chills; *comparison:* like a fireplace, oven, camp fire, sunshine, warm meal, slushy, stone, shade
- pressure—sharp, heavy, even, uneven, supportive, crushing, restricting, tight, pulsating, thud, throb
- weight—light, heavy, imbalanced, uneven, stuck
- tension—solid, dense, warm, cold, inflamed, protective, constricting, angry, sad, tight
- pain—ache, sharp, twinge, slight, stabbing, throbbing, dull, comes and goes
- tingling—pins and needles, prickly, vibration, tickling, numb
- size—small, large, huge, tiny
- shape—round, sharp, geometric, flat, circular, blob, mountainous
- motion—static, stationary, circular, erratic, straight, curved, gentle
- speed—fast, slow, still, slow motion
- texture—rough, wood, stone, sandpaper, smooth, silk, liquid
- element—fire, air, earth, water, wood
- color—opaque, gray, red, orange, etc.
- mood / emotion—sinking, drowning, running, pulling in, open, closed, uplifting, sunny day, dark cloud, inviting, shaming, shutting down, inflamed, raging, torrential
- sound—buzzing, singing, ringing, murmuring, humming
- taste—sour, bitter, sweet, salt, tangy
- smell—pungent, sweet, earthy, damp, like dog, like rain, like cut grass

- absence / nothingness—blank, empty, numb, nothing, hollow
- intensity—mild, strong, inconsistent

Describe these sensations out loud and allow yourself to fully feel them. It can be helpful to record yourself on a device during this process if you are alone. The purpose of saying them out loud is to be able to name them and potentially get to know them better the more often they appear. The purpose is not to change them (not at this stage anyway) but simply allow them to be present without judging or trying to alter them. Whether they register as pleasant or unpleasant, the challenge is in being able to stay present to them rather than block them, push them away, or get too attached or distracted by them. When we are able to let sensations arise within us and name them, we are better able to give them meaning, purpose, and understanding. We can better integrate them (like Lewis) to inform motivation: "Why do I have sex?" like we learned all about in chapter 6. In being better equipped to explore the process of embodiment in this way we make the potential to access pleasure and desire more available. Getting used to tuning in to the body allows us to be more aware of its responses to certain kinds of touch or stimulation, whether internal or external.

Try this activity for fifteen minutes a day, every day for a week. Notice what emerges each day and pay attention to any patterns or irregularities that you find as well as consistencies. All of this is great practice for tuning in to the impermanent nature of embodiment as a living, ever-changing being.

Zeroing In

An alternative to the scan is to choose one area at a time and see what emerges when you focus upon it. If you encounter a part of the body that elicits a traumatic or challenging response, do not panic. Place your hand on that part and send your breath to it using your imagination. Remind yourself you are safe and thank the sensation for showing itself. Do not force or press past what you are able to manage comfortably. You may not experience the same sensation every time in that part. Practicing allowing it to emerge is part of making room for embodiment to exist. If you begin to feel too much too soon, switch your attention to another part of your body. If that feels too much, stop. Take a glass of water and recalibrate. Try again another time.

If during zeroing you experience a sensation that is pleasant, neutral, or just plain curious, go into it further. You do this by sending breath to that place via your imagination and increasing the attention you place on it. As you breathe, feel that sensation becoming more magnified in whatever way that resonates for you. Don't worry about it "making sense." It most likely won't—at this stage anyway. We don't ask ourselves why we like the taste of something delicious, we just allow ourselves to enjoy it, so practice the same approach with exploring other sensations beyond taste. Just accept that it's a sensation that is pleasant. Describe it in as much detail as possible to a partner, friend or on your recording device. This allows you to be able to expand the sensation more fully and listen back to it for context and further understanding.

The Grounding Base Breath

Once you have been able to tune in to the body's sensations, you may like to practice amplifying or downplaying them. One of the most effective ways to do this is through breath. Breathing is integral to this practice whether at a beginner or advanced level. The Grounding Base Breath is really useful in helping connect to the body as it involves breathing in such a way that the entire torso and digestive tract is activated all the way from the mouth to the anus (which incidentally are the opposing ends of the exact same tube). Again, find a comfortable position, lying down if you can. Lying down on your back is useful as it forces you to breathe deeply into the lungs and not just shallow at a chest level. Place your feet flat on the floor with your knees bent. If this isn't possible, a chair is also fine, just remember to expand the lungs and belly as you breathe.

Breathe in, connect with the expanding balloon and this time imagine it (in your own way) expanding width ways as before and also length ways. As it expands down the length of your torso, imagine it gently pushing your pelvic floor muscles down and away from the body. Bear down slightly as if you were going to poop (but not so much that you do) and feel your anus puckering out ever so gently, as if it were "kissing" the surface beneath you. Allow yourself to connect with these deep sensations of the pelvic floor being tickled from the inside by your breath. I like to imagine the sound of Barry White's voice in my head for such activities. He knows how get deep, deep, deep, way down low. Then as you exhale, allow the air out of your mouth and feel the pelvic floor muscles and anus return to their regular state again.

Level Up

Once you have the hang of the sensation of breathing and bearing down slightly, try focusing your attention on a slightly exaggerated exhale. In through the nose and out through the mouth. It may be easier to connect with more heightened levels of sensation by exhaling through the mouth. Try and see what feels best for you.

The good thing about working with breath in accessing desire is it gives us something to focus on instead of the racing thoughts of the mind, which may be a distraction from sex and part of the brakes network. Exhaling stimulates the parasympathetic nervous system, which decreases how fast the heart beats, which in turn relaxes us. This is called a "down-regulating" breath as it decreases anxiety and stress within the body. Additionally, the anus is a region that is notoriously tight, and a place where a lot of emotion gets "stuck." It's an area associated with taboo and shame for many people and as a result, gets little attention from medical or even bodymind practitioners. Stress and anxiety have a strong relationship to the gut and the digestive system of which the anus is an important part. For many of us, stress and anxiety are centred around poor gut and anal function. Ever heard the expression "So-and-so is a tight-ass!" or "Such-and-such is so anal"? They're describing someone who is lacking in flexibility, openness, and spirit. While this may not be true literally, tightness in the anus and pelvic floor can stem from insecurity and a reflex to protect, fear and feeling unsafe enough to let go. Tightness in the pelvic floor and the anus in particular can be a hindrance to pleasure and desire and this technique is a gentle and non-invasive way to get this part of the body to soften, without feeling too confronting or exposing.

The Body Is the Home of Better Sex. Frankly!

Whether explicit trauma is present or not, learning to tune in to the body by imposing relaxation is helpful. Breath can control the brain's stress responses and our ability to control our physical responses.

Practicing "down regulating" breath and body techniques are useful for helping us tune in to the "felt sense," especially if there is a little bit of blockage or numbness. An "up-regulating" breath (which emphasizes the inhale), increases intensity and stimulation of the senses, so it's also useful for exaggerating what is present if we want to feel it more. Play with inhalations via the nose and the mouth and see how your body responds differently according to where oxygen enters. As a general rule, more air is taken in via the mouth than the nose. By increasing the amount of oxygen you take in during sex, you can feel more alive within your body. Learning to practice controlling sensations within your body can lead to feeling safer; which can in turn help create more pleasure and desire during sex.

In the next chapter we build on these foundational embodiment skills and, with your permission, level up to more explicit erotic practices. You may like to hang out with this chapter for a while longer before graduating to the next place, or you may like to skip over the explicit sexual stuff entirely. It's really up to you. Practice feeling your body and noticing how it responds to the options created in this book so far and moving forward. Because pleasure matters. Because what you want matters. And because the most important part of desire is honoring yourself in your quest to find it.

CHAPTER 9

~

Let's Get Physical

Not everything that is faced can be changed, but nothing can be changed until it is faced.

—James Baldwin

Until now, we have spent a lot of time exploring the concepts, emotions, and science that sit behind sex, libido, and pleasure, and how they relate to desire. In this chapter, we take these notions to the body and begin to explore *touch*, in addition to the embodiment practices we learned in the previous chapter, as the vehicle through which we can experience the erotic. This chapter is more activity-oriented (physical as well as reflective) than the previous ones, so you are invited to really pay attention to what your body is doing, feeling, and anticipating as you proceed through this chapter. We can feel anxious admitting to ourselves what we like and what we don't like when it comes to sex. And this can increase exponentially when we decide to admit it to someone else whose opinion matters to us. This chapter provides some suggestions to learn how to experiment with different kinds of touch for their own sake, if you would like to try them. Not everyone likes or wants partnered touch, so options are provided for exercises in solo contexts too. Allow yourself permission to find your own unique motivators for these activities, going back to your *why* in chapter 6, and then add them to your template as you discover what your body enjoys or yearns for. Go at your own speed and take breaks where necessary. It's essential to take the time to concentrate on what matters, especially if you are new to this process. One of the greatest causes of erotic anxiety and disconnect from desire is our discomfort with simply being with ourselves sexually, and discovering what is true and present in our lives.

So now—let's get practical.

One of the most basic forms of human connection is touch. For some of us it's hard to imagine life without it. From erotic passion to profound love—for some, but not all, of us—there is no deeper expression of affection, emotion, and eroticism. Sadly, many of us are touch-starved, not only because we don't touch, but because we don't know how to really give and receive touch. Seems absurd, doesn't it? After all, for some, touch is at the center of what "good sex" is about. But when was the last time you were touched in ways that rippled right through your body? In ways that left you yearning? In ways that left you feeling nourished and fulfilled? Many of us learn to tune out of sex because the touch we receive is not to our liking. We learn to tolerate touch we don't like, but then do not consider, What might make it better? How would we like to be touched instead? And then how do we say it?

Culturally speaking, it's complex navigation to tell someone we want to experience another kind of touch than what they are doing, especially if we don't want to hurt their feelings. Especially if we have tolerated it for years and to speak up now would be a real disruption. The implication is that we *should* enjoy the touch we get, no matter what. That we *should* be grateful someone wants to touch us—whether for our benefit or not.

Some of the biggest hurdles partners face in relationships are negotiating sex, pleasure, and intimacy. Who touches whom? How? When? Where? Often this nuance is skipped over entirely. The defaults tend to be touch as a means of leading to traditional sex rather than touch as an erotic experience of its own kind. So-called foreplay is intended to lead to penetration (particularly between heterosexual and gay male couples) with little emphasis on discussion, exploration, or determining who or what is being offered sexually, and who *exactly* is benefitting from the kind of sex on offer, and how. I say so-called foreplay because the implication behind the word is that it's the thing that comes before "something else" . . . even though the "something else" is rarely negotiated, all the activities preceding it imply it's the most likely outcome. But few of us stop to consider how we might make this different if we wanted to and what such consideration might make possible for desire to emerge, especially if ours is more responsive, like we learned in chapter 5.

The Wheel of Consent

Somatic sexologist Dr. Betty Martin has created a model of touch called the Wheel of Consent[1](see figure 9.1) that beautifully illustrates the mechanics of touch when, specifically, taking turns to bring our attention to *where* the pleasure is and *who* it's for. This model is

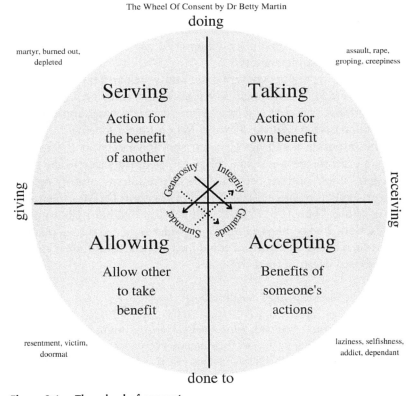

Figure 9.1. The wheel of consent.
Source: Betty Martin. B. Martin, and R. Dalzen. *The Art of Receiving and Giving: The Wheel of Consent* (Eugene, OR: Luminare Press, 2021).

brilliant in helping us identify that, in short, the person *doing the touching* is not always the person *doing the giving*, while the recipient of the touch is not always *being pleasured*. Martin's theory proposes that in any instance of touch, there are two powerful factors: *who's doing it?* and *who it's for*. Those two factors combine in a variety of ways that encompass the *serve, take, allow,* and *accept* quadrants.

Each quadrant presents its own challenges, lessons, and joys. Working with this model in this turn-taking fashion is helpful because it invites us to step out of the "business-as-usual" model of sex and touching. Most of us believe that for sex to be satisfying it must be mutually beneficial. And while that's true, the implication is it needs to be *simultaneously* beneficial, a much harder, and less likely expectation to meet. Instead, the Wheel of Consent Model invites us to *really* consider what we are doing in our sex practices and what our intentions are in doing so. This in turn gives us the framework to refer back to *why* we are having sex in the first place (chapter 6) and see if our "what" and our "why" are complementary.

The circle represents consent (you and your partner's agreement). Inside the circle, there is a gift given and a gift received. Outside the circle (without consent), the exact same action becomes unpleasant at best and abusive, violating at worst. When touch is being performed and the intention is not agreed upon and understood, it is often the cause of much distress in sexual relationships or the place where eroticism gets "stuck" and sex becomes boring, painful, or unsatisfying.

In an explicit practice of the Wheel of Consent, Dr. Martin encourages us to ask, "May I . . . ?" and "Will you . . . ?" rather than assuming what action is to be engaged. If we consider how a kiss may play out within each of the quadrants, it could look like the following, including the proposed questioning technique:

Taking (*Receiving* and *Doing* Halves)

"May I kiss you?" And with permission you charge on in, lips ready for action and pressing up against their mouth, you go for it as the focus of the practice is determined by you taking exactly what you want. Mutuality may not be the focus, although permission (either verbal or physical) is essential.

Allowing (*Giving* and *Done-to* Halves)

"May I kiss you?" you are asked. You respond affirmatively and open your mouth to receive the kiss that is presented. You participate in the kiss, allowing it to happen and may find it pleasurable too, or you are willing to participate wholeheartedly because it's something you know your partner enjoys.

Accepting (*Done-to* and *Receiving* Halves)

"Will you kiss me?" You ask your partner to kiss you and they respond with sensitivity and enthusiasm. You move yourself closer, showing approval with your moans or physical gestures, and signal to your partner how you like it, either through action or verbally.

Serving (*Doing* and *Giving* Halves)

"Will you kiss me?" you partner asks, and upon your agreement your kiss proceeds gently and softly, checking that what you are doing and how you are doing it is the same as what they had in mind. As you continue, you may stop to verbally check in how they are experiencing it, and they may respond with how fabulous it is and that they want more, deeper, or even harder. You agree, and continue to honor their request.

The purpose of this practice is multilayered. In the first instance, it provides a framework to help us talk explicitly about sex and get used to engaging in inquiry—both with ourselves and our partners—about what we are doing and the degree to which we are doing it. It invites us to make explicit who benefits from the interaction and who, *exactly*, it is for. It shows us how traditional "active" and "passive" interactions are actually far more nuanced and complex than simply giving and receiving, and it provides a framework for us to check in with ourselves about what's happening and how we feel about it. While in its pure form, some couples may balk at asking about something like kissing, it's a wonderful practice to experiment with as a means of discovering new things about your partner's sexual preferences that you perhaps had never known, despite the number of years together, and a wonderful thing to do with a new partner to help make sex richer and more fulfilling.

The Three Minute Game

A great way to practice this technique in a deeper way, or as a means to igniting your bodily responses, is with something Dr. Martin calls the "Three-Minute Game." In this you and your partner / friend *take turns* (this part is crucial) asking these two questions of each other:

1. How would you like *me* to touch *you* for three minutes? (The gift recipient might respond with: "Will you scratch my back, kiss my neck, bite my toes, hold me?" etc.)
2. How would *you* like to touch *me* for three minutes? (The gift recipient might respond with: "May I feel your arms, explore your back, play with your hair?" etc. This gift is for the doer's pleasure.)

Players negotiate the right amount of detail for the job and proceed for the duration of three minutes. Then take turns reversing roles until both people have experienced both roles.

Looking back at the model, the solid arrows in the center of the circle indicate who is *doing* the action, while the dotted arrows indicate who the gift is for, which is not always the person who is being done-to. In other words, the solid arrows show which way the action is going and the dotted arrows show which way the gift is going. Both offers come from the giving half and both requests come from the receiving half. Therefore, if you make the offer, you are giving a gift in both cases. Negotiate as needed. Never give more than you are happy to give.

If you'd like to try it, it's helpful to go slowly and to start with "non-sexy" areas, especially if sex brings up a little anxiety for you or your relationship, until you get a sense of the possibilities and challenges the game creates. Like describing pizza to someone who's never eaten it, it's hard to describe the flavor of touch and negotiating without trying it, so these following practices are really best as activities you do rather than concepts you imagine. Fulfillment comes from the agreements you create between you, about the kind of touch being offered and received and following who it's *for*. In being clear about who is doing the action *and* who is receiving the gift, it creates a new framework within which pleasure from touch can be defined, agreed on, and negotiated.

Agreements are embedded within the structure of the Three-Minute Game and even though such a process may feel clunky at the beginning, it's a helpful model to use to allow conversations about the physical aspects of touch to begin.

It's not uncommon for partners to rely upon good intentions for sex to "work out," but UK-based somatic sex educator Meredith Reynolds asks, "How reliable are such intentions when they require so much interpretation?" Instead, they suggest we:

> Agree the right level of detail for agreements. For some people, careful negotiation of details, before and during may be very important. For others, agreements about very significant activities mixed with "tuning in" for much of the time will feel right. And for some, a "go with the flow" approach may feel best, with an agreement to be honest with each other if something doesn't feel good. Be prepared to change, even if you had an agreement. Something that seemed a great idea earlier may not feel great right now, and an agreement is not a contract! Agree to be as honest as possible about what's working and what isn't.

Time for Reflection

How did it feel to explore the quadrants and practice the Three-Minute Game? Reading about it is one thing, but doing it allows us to really get intimate with what happens within us during partnered touch.

How did the Three-Minute Game interact with the values and conditions that you explored in chapter 6? Was it easy to ask for what you want? Was it easy to think about who the gift was for? What challenges presented themselves to you? Did you notice any familiar feelings emerge as you engaged in the practice? The more you discover about yourself and your pleasures, the more you can add to defining and refining your erotic template. Add this information to your notebook and revisit the game and the reflections as often as you like.

Case Study: Dante
When given the opportunity to really reflect on how we receive touch, it's interesting to note that while we often know when we're experiencing something we aren't enjoying, we might not know what to ask for or how to change it.

For example, Dante knew that she didn't like the way her girlfriend did oral sex. For Dante, it was too intense and she wanted something different. The trouble for Dante was she couldn't say what she preferred because she didn't know how to put it into words. In the past, she'd had really satisfying experiences of receiving oral sex that worked for her, but none of her prior partners had described what they were doing and it didn't occur to her to ask. So while she knew there *were* things she liked, she had no framework for saying it because she had no idea what they did that felt so good. In order to counter this, I often encourage clients to create "pleasure labs" as part of their regular erotic practice. The intention behind pleasure labs is not about having orgasms and getting off, although it's totally welcome. Instead, the purpose is to discover which techniques feel good, creating room for both partners to approach the lab from a place of curiosity, willingness, and priority (the Triangle of Satisfaction) to gain valuable information rather than driving a performance-oriented sex session. Part of their lab involved trying out different oral moves, and her only responsibility was to rate them on a pleasure scale of 1 to 10. These labs are powerful practices because they help us tune in to what we like, and since sensations can change when we're turned on, they practice the techniques during different states of arousal to work out what felt best and when.

In Dante's case they discovered that she liked light circles on her clitoris to start, and that she liked suction, but only when she was more warmed up. With this useful knowledge, she was able to let her girlfriend know when she was ready to change from softer to more intense stimulation, and her partner was more likely to be able to offer what she wanted. For Dante this was a breakthrough, because she'd never before known what she liked and thus how to ask for it. The power embedded in being able to say, "Make little circles on my clit," in contrast with, "Do that thing you did that time," is a game changer for many who traditionally don't know what they like or how they want to be touched.

Embodied Touch

After experimenting with the Three-Minute Game and the Wheel of Consent, you may be ready to amp it up a little in terms of experimenting with the kind of touch you like, and perhaps even kinds of touch you might like to give and receive with another. Embodied touch is an expressive way of integrating the body with the mind and emotions to create more intentional connection and perhaps more passion, potency and pleasure to your sexual expression. When we place our *attention* on our *intention*, we come closer into alignment with our *personal* values and conditions. The emphasis is on exploring sensation for its own sake, not on trying to race to the finish line, create an orgasm, desire for penetrative sex, or even anything that resembles what we might think of as traditional sex. And embodied touch is not just about *giving touch* for the benefit of the receiver with clear intention, focus, and awareness but also purposely *receiving touch* with the same intention and clarity. In other words, remaining aware of not only how you're feeling in the receiving role but also what you are *experiencing* physically in your partner's hands.

It's easy to mistakenly think that receiving touch in an intimate context is like receiving a professional massage; you can just drift away and zone out. It's easy to forget where we are or what we are doing in many of life's activities, like eating, driving, on public transport, on social media. Our lives are geared to make us zone out, especially when we are overworked and overstimulated. But sadly, disconnections and misunderstandings between giver and receiver, doer and taker are often the cause of erotic breakdowns between partners. Because most of us have never really learned or experienced the wonder of deeply connected and meaningful touch, we may not even know it exists. If we don't learn it at school and we don't see it on TV or in the movies, there is little chance we'll ever encounter it. We may have learned to emphasize touch in our homes growing up, but even this is rare. We simply don't live in a world that values it or knows how to explore it. Instead, we forget what our bodies need, or we never inquire and never know how exquisite erotic connection through simple touch can really be.

Mindful Self-Pleasure Practice

To begin, set your space just right for you. Consider the items on your erotic conditions list from chapter 6—things like lighting, textures in the room, fragrances, safety from prying eyes, music, and so on. Do you want to wear clothes? Be naked? Take the time to make things just so.

When you are ready, turn on some music with a medium tempo and take a minute or two to shake your whole body. Everything from your hair to your toes. Move with intention and just enough vigor to raise your heart rate a little, but not so much that speech would be difficult. Allowing your body to shake helps release tension, relaxes the mind, and softens the muscles. After settling, decide if you'd like to do this practice sitting, lying down, or perhaps standing if that's your preferred stance. When settled, bring awareness to your breath and the rise and fall of your chest and abdomen. Notice any sensations, feelings, or thoughts that arise with softness and curiosity. Tune in to your heart and your heartbeat. Place your right hand over your heart, making a loop from your heart to your shoulder, down your arm to your hand, and back to your heart. Linger a moment and resist the temptation to race ahead should it arise. Don't be surprised if you experience deep waves of pleasure and sensation from this process alone.

When you're ready, with any hand, touch your arm. Focus on the sensation of what the hand and fingers can feel first. Then switch your attention to the arm—the recipient of the touch. How does that part feel being touched? What kinds of sensations does it long for? Firm, long strokes? Light, feathery touch? Pinching, thudding, or stinging? Try a variety of sensations. Practice asking your body what *feels* best and be curious with it, offering it the sensations it seems to respond to. Notice how it responds, including changes in skin color, temperature, sensitivity, and so on. Continue to shift your awareness to different parts of your body that are touching or being touched, respectively (remembering to focus on touching *or* being touched, but not both at the same time).

If you are ready to explore more than the arms, set an intention for the self-touch experience. It may be something like permission: "My intention is to experience pleasure for its own sake without shame"; or, "to experience a different kind of erotic sensation—do something out of my normal masturbation routine"; or maybe, "to experience masturbation without ejaculation." Allow yourself to engage in a self-touch ritual or masturbation practice, but instead of doing what you would always do (assuming you do masturbate), with the same toys, techniques, or porn, try different techniques and positions, move your body instead of being still, breathe in and out more intentionally, just to see how your body responds. If masturbation is not something you do very often, perhaps you'd like to try it out now? The focus is not on orgasm, but simply on touching with awareness just to see what happens. We are allowing our bodies to guide us with the sensations being the locus of our attention. Take as much time as you like, being aware that it can often take at least twenty minutes for the mind and body to begin to connect, especially if we spend most of our days thinking and getting stuff done.

Complete the experience as you like, thanking your body for showing up for you and allowing you to experience its pleasure.

Take some time to reflect on what your body enjoyed and write about it in your notebook. How long did it take before it started to feel erotic? Perhaps it didn't feel erotic and instead felt something else? What was enjoyable about the experience? What was difficult?

What sensations did your body enjoy that surprised you? What sensations did your body enjoy that you knew about? How might this knowledge inform your erotic template including what you might ask a partner for in terms of sex, when knowing what your body likes as well as what your brain values and heart wants?

Mindful Erotic Massage for Couples

As lovers, we often try to touch and be touched at the same time. This notion of mutual, simultaneous pleasure is rife in Western culture. While it's a great idea, in reality, it's not often mutual and it's not always pleasurable, for at least one party. It's hard to both give *and* receive touch simultaneously with full awareness. As an alternative, I propose focusing on the pleasure of one person at a time, to practice giving and receiving touch intentionally. In this instance, practice through the vehicle of erotic massage. Studies have shown[2] that when we give and receive touch with intention, we are able to communicate more effectively and intuitively than with words alone.

Like the solo practice, consider what you need to make things just right. Sights, sounds, smells, door locks, perhaps a massage table if you have one, or a surface where both masseur and recipient can be comfortable for a sustained period of time. Consider towels, sheets, pillows, and any oils you may like to use for the massage including the temperatures of the oils and the room itself. It's remarkable how many people skip over the comfort part to get to the touch part, but in the end, the lack of comfort derails the whole experience for both parties. If this will include genital massage, do you have your preferred toys (etc.) readily at hand? Are they clean? Charged? And compatible with your chosen oil or lubricant? Once settled, ask the receiver to lie facedown on the massage table or bed. Invite them to focus on their breath, to invite relaxation, and perhaps set an intention for the massage: "Is there anywhere you don't want to be touched?" This sets clear boundaries about what is off limits for this session. A simple response could be, "I don't want any penetration vaginally or anally, but I do want clitoral touch." Receivers can state (verbally) what they would like—sensual touch, arousing touch, genital touch, basic massage—activating the taking / accepting half of the wheel. Givers can bring all of their attention to this request to offer the kind of touch requested, or an alternative all parties are comfortable with. This matches with the "serving" quadrant of Martin's Wheel of Consent Model.

The person being touched doesn't need to justify or explain their response. Just as we don't justify *why* we want a certain touch, we don't need to justify why we *don't* want something. A simple "thank you" on the part of the toucher indicates, "I have heard you and I won't be touching you there." When they are ready to receive touch, they can let you know.

Introduce your touch, initially, by simply holding still. It can be nice to begin with one hand on the back of their heart and the other on their lower back. Be still and synchronize your breath. Then massage one side of the back, using long, firm, gliding strokes to apply oil. Remember this is sensual massage, not remedial or sports massage. Don't dig in. Instead, turn-on and awaken. Many people enjoy broad circular strokes over the back. Press into the muscles along the spine with your hands flat, but do not create pressure on the spine itself.

Invite the person receiving guide you rather than zoning out. Ask them specific questions like:

- Would more or less pressure feel better here?
- Would faster or slower feel better there?

Touch one side of the back and then the other, including the shoulders, with kneading strokes to help release a little pressure and tension. Complete with long, gliding strokes over both sides of the back, starting from the head all the way down to the sacrum. Return to the original side of your massage and, with their permission, move to the butt cheek. Start with stillness, then slow gentle circles, increasing the speed and pressure as you invite feedback. Remember this is about active receiving, not zoning out for a nap. Continue down the legs one side of the body at a time, with gliding strokes and adequate oil, mindful of not putting pressure on their knees. Experiment with different kinds of sensation to awaken the body, as well as relax it. Feathery stroking, scratches, thuds, slaps, and tapping can all be enjoyable. Discover and communicate.

When inviting them to turn over, be mindful of the inherent vulnerability in revealing one's belly. For humans, as in the animal world, the tender underside is significant emotionally, socially, and viscerally. Move slowly and deliberately; let them settle. Position yourself behind their head to work the shoulders and chest area including nipples and breast / chest tissue as they like it, on all genders, with consent. Massage the neck and face from this position also, though with limited oil on the face. Move to one side of their body to include the arm, hand, and fingers, then down the front of the leg, again avoiding pressure on the knee. The fullness of our thighs can enjoy long, strong, deep gliding strokes and well as wringing strokes. Repeat all this on the other side and remember to invite feedback all the while: "What would make this better?"; "What would you like more of?"; and so forth. If you are integrating genital touch, start slowly, intentionally, and with the sensitivity addressed in the Wheel of Consent and the Three-Minute Game. (See the resources on my website for more explicit and detailed descriptions of erotic massage techniques.) Do only what was agreed and avoid adding any more activities without negotiation, at this stage anyway. This is where the practice of continued and deliberate interaction makes the experience of intentional embodied touch so different from a sleepy massage or sex where we just take what we are given, whether we like it or not. With this formula you get to practice saying what you want. Hearing what is and is not wanted. Tolerating the challenge of not giving what you want to give. Honoring what is requested and only that, all while paying attention to how their body and your body respond to touch and what that might mean for your erotic template. Additionally, we can consider what could help you ease the brakes, if required, and what, if anything, might increase the gas a little.

After the massage, take some time to reflect on your experience, whether masseur or recipient. Again, pay attention to things like how your body responded and write this information down. It's vital content for knowing how to incorporate the body into your exploration of desire and your erotic template.

There is a lot the body and especially touch can teach us about our desires and how they connect to our thoughts and feelings. In chapter 4, we learned about Basson's circular human sexuality model, which suggests that desire may well live in the body before it even registers with the mind (an idea also supported by the notion of responsive desire). By learning to allow the body to guide us a little, spending time taking turns exploring, recognizing that pleasure is idiosyncratic and highly individualized, tolerating the discomfort and ambiguity of our bodies, and creating time and space for our bodies to reveal themselves to us, we create new possibilities for pleasure and, perhaps, desire to emerge. All this takes time, patience, practice, willingness, and, ultimately, just enough risk to examine parts of our eroticism that are obscured by a lack of information and education. The information you discovered about your responses to the Wheel of Consent, the Three-Minute Game, the solo touch /masturbation practice, and the partnered erotic massage (if you had the opportunity to try it) are all prized knowledge for your erotic template. Knowing what you like, what you want, and how to ask for it are some of the most valuable tools you will ever learn. In the next chapter, we dive into the role of risk-taking as a tool for accessing desire and discovering even more wisdom for our erotic template before moving on to learning how to communicate about sex with those who we most need to share this with.

CHAPTER 10

~

Taking Risks

I had everything I needed except the courage to admit that I was
the one holding the door, playing with the keys.

—Susie Bright

Risk-taking is often associated with adrenaline, danger, and impulsive
or bad decision-making. It's linked to courage and creativity in professional pursuits but to peril and a lack of self-control when explored in
sexuality. While risk-taking is permitted—even expected—for men
(sexual risks are deemed dangerous and stupid, yet if you don't take
them, you're not a real man), it is still categorically discouraged for
everyone else.

In my research for this chapter, many of the articles I found about
sexual risk-taking reinforced ideas of danger, reckless behavior, and a
lack of care and regard for one's self and partners, and blamed it for
increases in STI transmission. While those aspects are real, there is
a glaring omission in the clinical literature about the value of erotic
risk-taking and the benefit of its engagement on passion and desire.
Its exclusion suggests that risk-taking is not important or worthy but,
rather, mere folly.

When it comes to sexual satisfaction, nothing could be further from the truth. In order to create a more fulfilling relationship with sexuality and ultimately desire, it is essential that we look at the obvious and hidden forces at work that prevent risk-taking from being addressed constructively. By making the implicit explicit, we edge closer to taking back our eroticism from the no-go zones we habitually avoid. This is expertly articulated by one of my best friends and mentors Barbara Carrellas as follows:

> Without risk, there is no growth or energy; however, without support, risk becomes recklessness. In the territory between, we can grow, thrive, and find pleasure.[1]

Western culture has a strong attachment to certainty. We are obsessed with the idea that every problem has a solution. We like our solutions to be clearly laid out, with neither ambiguity nor any need for interpretation. We minimize risk to reduce our feelings of insecurity and inadequacy. Outcomes are defined so that we can measure ourselves against them.

This is reinforced by sexual health medicine's focus on sexual function and dysfunction, often reducing sex to a basic set of repetitive practices. If these practices fail, take a pill and work harder until sex "works" again. Medicine doesn't consider exploring alternatives or discussing what turns you on, how your body responds to pleasure, or how to manage the stigma or erotic vulnerability. If you can't do sex the conventional way, then you've failed and it's not *real* sex—it's merely "foreplay," is the line we're fed. The implication of traditional medical narratives is that men are hardwired for emotionless sex and must have erections for sex to be fulfilling, while women get aroused by romance, intimacy, and watching men do housework. Never mind the people whose sexuality or gender sits outside of this limitation. For most of us, it's "fuck or get fucked"; and not in a way that we enjoy.

In chapter 5 we looked at the role the brain plays in helping us organize basic emotions that inform our sexual practices, like fear and excitement. We also had an introduction to the Dual Control Model and how the SES (our sexual excitement system that operates like a gas pedal in a car) and SIS (our sexual inhibition system that operates like the brakes) help us understand how our sexual expression functions in our day-to-day lives. While such scales and emotions are helpful in determining the context of understanding ourselves, we also know from clinical research including the brain science that such considerations are not hardwired but are developed in response to circumstances and experiences. This suggests that what has been learned can be unlearned and replaced with responses more aligned with how we'd *like* to experience sex. As we discovered in chapters 6 through 9, we are so much more than just our brains, so making connections between our thoughts, values, emotions, bodies, embodied touch, and arousal are all vital factors that can help us shift our visceral experiences of desire to be more in alignment with how we want to want sex, if indeed we do.

Taking erotic risks can be about engaging in new sex practices or, more importantly, about doing something different and invigorating. Changing the environment, changing the routine, or changing the focus are all examples of taking risks. Even the Dual Control Model asks us to consider what makes us put our foot on the brakes, in order to risk taking our foot off a little. For a sexual risk to be of benefit, regardless of the outcome, there needs to be an element of purpose and enthusiasm behind it.

But the courage to take sexual risks is more nuanced than thrill seeking for its own sake. For some of us, risk-taking comes easily, but for others, it's an invitation to tune in to not only what we want but also to what prevents us being closer to ourselves, our desires, or our longings. Finding support for such processes is essential. One of my great teachers, the late Chester Mainard, described the reticence to move toward risk and take our foot off the brake, as a manifestation of sexual shame. He explains it thusly:

> One of the tricky things about shame is that it is often invisible to the person experiencing it. Shame creates an "electric fence" within ourselves. Once you get shocked two or three times you stay back from the fence. The electricity can get turned off but you still don't go near the fence anymore. When we are operating in our comfort zone, we are actually operating inside the shame. Shame operates by avoiding the feeling

of it, and it's tricky sometimes to notice what you are avoiding. "Oh, I'm not feeling anything right now." That may be true, or maybe shame is operating so well that you've learned to stay well inside that fence, not taking any risks that may result in the activation of the shame.

For some people, the risks involved in sex are not physical but emotional. Avoiding the electric fence and keeping a foot on the brake has become so ingrained that we no longer notice it. It feels "normal," but it also no longer acts as protection but, rather, inhibition. And while inhibition serves a great purpose in preventing us from making mistakes or hurting ourselves or others, it does not necessarily foster self-reflection. Instead, it demands attention by shutting connection down completely.

Erotic risks look different to different people. For those who seek adventures, a risk may entail experiencing the vulnerability of intimacy. For someone for whom sex always happens "externally" (i.e., doing the penetrating), a risk may be exploring the sensations of being penetrated. For someone for whom sex mostly happens internally (i.e., being penetrated), a risk may be experiencing the exquisite intensity of doing the penetrating. For someone who is accustomed to having an erection during sex, a risk might be allowing themselves to be seen or touched while soft. For someone for whom initiating sex feels confronting, taking the time to invite a partner to pleasure might be experienced as a risk.

The possibilities of risk-taking are essentially endless.

Although we know that people who score higher on the SES are more likely to take risks sexually than those scoring higher on the SIS, it's unclear how emotional risk-taking relates to people scoring highly on either scale. Most studies have been limited in measuring individual differences such as emotional adaptation to vulnerability and sexual shame. Regardless, current evidence describing the impact of emotional regulation on well-being informs us that, when practiced regularly, paying attention to our electric fences and our brakes network may strengthen our "emotional muscles," which in turn can counteract the effects of past experiences and may even prevent future sexual difficulties.

Case Study: Mel and Chris
Mel and Chris are a queer-identified couple. Mel identifies as gender queer and uses "they / them" pronouns while Chris uses "she / her." Mel and Chris first came to see me with a strong relationship but a dissatisfying sex life. Both were smart, kind, and happy with their relationship but felt stuck in a hole they couldn't escape.

While they both had broad experience in sexual practices, they were not each other's first or only partners and had previously enjoyed a rich array of activities from "vanilla" practices (things that are usually referred to as "normal" genitally-based sex) through to exploring kinkier and rougher practices including bondage, power play, and rough sex.

The sex problem was often experienced by both of them as a fraught sexual disconnection. Sex became a loaded issue. It was difficult to talk about and processing the weighty implications of what they were and were not doing sexually often took precedence over simply getting on with doing it.

While communication is an essential cornerstone of effective erotic practice, in the case of Mel and Chris it seemed that too much of a good thing was a libido killer. By the time they got to me they were both pretty "over-processed." The eroticism they longed for failed to flourish under the weight of rigorous emotional analysis and interpretation, and relentless inquiry.

Mel, although having what they called a "high libido"—meaning they wanted sex more frequently than Chris—struggled to express their eroticism in ways that made them feel confident and good about themself.

"I know what I like," Mel said, "but I just feel I am too much for Chris."

"It's not that you're too much," Chris retorted with compassion yet resignation, "but this neediness is too much. You're not too much but *it* is really too much."

Chris sighed and looked down at the floor. She knew what she had said would be hard to hear, but it was a truth that had to be spoken.

Despite the intensity of such a comment, it was essential that Mel really got what Chris was saying: Mel wasn't too much but the intense neediness was. I could see Mel was crestfallen and I wanted to point out that what Chris had said was not a criticism, just a fact.

"Mel, did you hear that Chris said *you* are not the problem but the *intensity* is?"

"Huh?" Mel looked at me glassy-eyed. "What do you mean?"

"It's not your wanting sex that is the issue here, but rather your discomfort with that. That's what unnerves Chris."

Chris was nodding. "Yes, yes, yes . . . I like sex too and I want it but when we don't have it, it doesn't mean I think you're too much . . . this is hard for me too, you know."

Slowly, we were getting to the core of the issue. What seemed initially like a desire discrepancy was proving to be something more. They had different needs, but it didn't seem to be just a desire problem.

I invited them to attend individual counseling sessions to get to the bottom of it. Sometimes speaking to couples separately allows them to talk frankly about sex without accidentally offending the other person.

Mel attended their solo session first. Despite their sexual maturity and experience, Mel often felt inadequate and unable to satisfy Chris. As a teen, Mel found that sex was an invigorating experience and, while not exploring "queerness" explicitly from that age, they were attracted to a wide variety of people and engaged in "a lot of sex" with "a lot of people." Over time, Mel was shamed and humiliated for this robust exploration, and experienced feelings of shame because of the fluid that would appear in their underwear. Too sexual, too aroused, and simply too much, Mel felt that their sexuality needed to be reined-in in order to be acceptable. This created a chasm—an electric fence between what they experienced emotionally and what they wanted to do physically—so they began to shut communication down.

For many of us, our emotional experiences as children and teenagers can have a profound effect on how we express ourselves sexually as adults. These experiences needn't be erotic as such, nor even cases of abuse or molestation, but, rather, explorations of sensual, emotional, and sexual needs going unmet, unfulfilled, or unresolved that creep into our sexual relationships as adults. Unsettled emotions from this developmental time can and often do have an impact many years later and, while way outside the realm of the rational mind of logic and reason, are a powerful force that can manifest in unhelpful ways. Smart, educated, and cognizant people may still struggle with such unresolved inner conflicts. As we learned earlier, such raw emotions and sexuality can impact us in ways that transcend the "logical" brain by creating an electric fence that separates us from ourselves, even when the electricity is turned off. In other words, even though we realize it's not what we want, we still find ourselves avoiding the fence. This discomfort can lead us to shut down and not take risks for fear of reactivating old wounds and painful memories or sensations.

Even though Mel knew Chris didn't think *they* were too much, the sense of shame was engulfing for them. It's a rare person who hasn't experienced discomfort around what they want and how they behave, especially when it comes to sex. Despite our logical mind telling us differently, old beliefs persist. In some cases, the experience of being shamed for our body, our identity, or our way of being sexual, can have repercussions that can crop up as adults and affect otherwise great relationships. The experience of feeling "too much" meant expression was dangerous, especially when Mel didn't know if they would be received or rejected by Chris. This manifested as an awkwardness and a clumsiness with touch and sexual activities that made the once-enthusiastic Mel feel like an inexperienced sexual novice.

During her individual session, Chris told me that in the relationship with Mel she was doing much of the emotional work—managing the sadness of not enough sex, talking about the shame of being too much, and initiating conversations when the silences became too cold. Chris knew that emotions were a part of any relationship, but when this was conflated with Mel's neediness, that acted as a libido killer for Chris. Sex was the last thing on her mind after a heavy conversation, processing emotions. Being compelled to take a management role within the emotional side of the relationship, meant that Chris found it hard to switch her brain into "sexy mode" and "go-with-the-flow," which is how she used to experience herself sexually. While she trusted Mel with her life, she didn't trust them with their capacity to be self-soothing and receptive during sex. This left Chris feeling hypervigilant and unable to relax into sexual play. The fear was that Mel would become overwhelmed during sex and simply abandon the play, leaving Chris high-and-dry and feeling disconnected from Mel, retreating back into feeling overwhelmed by shame. That was a risk Chris was not prepared to take without some reassurance that Mel was able to take a bit more care of themself and their emotions, particularly during sex.

It turned out that what Chris most wanted was to be able to surrender sexually. During sex, she simply wanted to be able to experience abandon. She wanted to be ravished, taken, and held at Mel's discretion. But she needed to be sure Mel was up for it. Chris didn't want to have to coach Mel through "top" sex, as well as their complex emotional shame, so instead she did nothing.

With neither wanting to hurt each others' feelings, yet both deeply dissatisfied, it became apparent that finding ways to explore sex, power, and surrender—without having to explicitly discuss its implications—was required. Too many meaty conversations and too much emotional processing had rendered them removed from their playfulness and joy.

In queer circles and communities, there is a lot of discussion about the lack of visibility of queer sexuality and sexual practices in broader culture. Like the erasure of risk-taking's value, this sexual omission implies that queerness is not necessarily bad but, essentially, not valuable. Mainstream romance novels and movies tend to depict mostly straight and heterosexual couples doing fairly "straight" things, with little attention paid to depictions of sex outside this, regardless of the genders of the people involved. Because most of us do not get the opportunity to see others engaging in sex with the same liberty, we get to see how others paint, cook, or play music, it can be hard to re-imagine sex without external references. "Spice It Up," the advice columns all say; but what does that mean if we've never seen nor experienced it before? How do you describe curry to someone who's never tasted it? The limitations in our sexual menus are reinforced when depictions of sex are always focused on intercourse. While we wait for Hollywood narratives to start portraying more frequent, authentic, and diverse sexual expression (even among heterosexuals), one group of filmmakers have already heeded the call. In response to this glaring omission, some contemporary pornographers are recognizing the need for diversity from an entertainment point of view, at a minimum, but, when done well, such material can also be useful, creative, inspirational, and therapeutic.

After a discussion with Chris and Mel about using porn (and gaining consent from both of them to proceed), I referred them to the online Crash Pad Series[2] as a source of erotic motivation, to not only trigger their imaginations but also create a template through which they could explore more useful sexual motivations to kick start their sex life again. Crash Pad Series is a website that provides visual media content that specializes in queer identities and a broad diversity of erotic dynamics beyond just "vanilla." The performers create "scenes," on their own terms, and film themselves in the privacy of their unique "crash pad." The intimacy and intensity depicted in these clips is often palpable and far more curated and involved than the high intensity / low intimacy scenes we tend to think of in more conventional porn. I was curious if they could gain some traction by using their discovery of the content of this site as a catalyst to discuss their preferences and explore new kinds of eroticism. Because of its diversity, I hoped Chris could find representations of sex that she found exciting, and Mel could augment their toolbox of skills based on what Chris said she found to be a turn on.

The Crash Pad Series experiment yielded tremendous results for them. Within a few weeks the pair were relishing sex on their terms, inspired by what they had seen, were communicating better (by their standards) and felt closer overall. Chris initially found a few scenes she liked, depicting either acts or power dynamics that she wanted to experience. With Mel's permission they watched these together and used them as inspiration for creating their own erotic scenes. Because Chris chose them, Mel understood that these were scenes that appealed to her. This was a crucial part in the success of this experiment, because Chris got to ask for what she wanted without having to use words. And Mel was able to enter into sex with Chris feeling more confident, as they already knew what Chris liked and was hoping for. Mel was no longer required to second guess themself and was able to express the full passion of their sexuality, and to even take control, knowing that Chris was enjoying and relishing the full encounter. Chris was able to relax into the surrendering role she longed for, feeling more confident that Mel would be able to go the distance and not become overwhelmed by emotion. By minimizing endless complex conversations and clunky emotional processing, they took a risk with their sexual activity. Their focus was on pleasure rather than habit or staying behind the electric fence. With the Triangle of Satisfaction firmly established for support, the pair were able to move through to the next stage of their erotic relationship with fulfilment and confidence on their side.

Setting the Stage for Risk-Taking

When you are taking a risk sexually, you needn't be overly enthusiastic but you do need to be engaged in the process. Obstacles can be aphrodisiacs, as we have discovered with the Erotic Equation (chapter 3), so engaging with supported risk-taking in sex can be a real erotic boost, just like for Mel and Chris. It's a matter of determining *where I am* in contrast with *where I would like to get*. Waiting for everything to be perfect can function as an excuse to stay in your comfort zone.

Dr. Betty Martin, the creator of the Wheel of Consent from the previous chapter, suggests there are ways we can "allow" such experiences, should we find the motivation—much like the first time we take a plane trip, attend a job interview—like Mel and Chris did with porn, or anything else where the *incentive* is informed by the *reward*. We may be unsure of the outcome, but the consequences of *not* doing it, are far worse.

Sometimes getting stuck sexually is the result of shutting down imagination and inspiration. In *Mating in Captivity*, author Esther Perel suggests this is the source of sex that has become curtailed, devoid of vibrancy and ultimately boring.[3] Whether it's dependent upon taking inspiration from using porn like Mel and Chris, erotic literature, blogs, sex classes, or just getting creative with sex and having fun, taking sexual risks requires preparation. With this in mind, it's essential we move forward with one of the cornerstones of the Triangle of Satisfaction (from chapter 7) in mind: curiosity. Just like sitting at a bus stop, there are few situations in life where we would expect to arrive at our destination without making a move of some kind. Practicing taking risks with our sexuality and interests demands that our bodies act as a vehicle to free us from the limitations of a fenced-off state of mind. When our minds are out of sync with our physical sensations and desires, it's difficult to find motivation and enthusiasm for change.

Acclaimed neurology expert Dan Siegel reminds us that, if change is indeed what we seek, we can work more effectively by altering unhelpful emotional pathways through using the body rather than by simply discussion alone.[4] This may explain why Mel and Chris felt so bogged down with their endless discussions and needed action to create change.

Time for Reflection

Allow time to daydream and imagine yourself in the "most fulfilling" erotic scenario. These are not things you necessarily need to do or act out. Just allow the feelings and ideas to emerge without shame, judgement, or turning away from them.

- How would you like to feel during sex? What would you try if you knew you could not "fail"?
- If you could put what you really wanted on a microchip and insert it into the mind of your partner (current or future) without having to say it out loud, what would it be?
- What would you like your partner (current or future) to know about your erotic preferences?

(Don't mind how you say it at this stage, we'll be looking at that later—just get the idea out of your head and down on paper.)

Notice how it feels to not only think such thoughts but also to stick with them long enough to write them down. Remember that paying attention to our feelings and physical sensations in this way is part of getting used to them. Allowing them to surface, despite any discomfort, is part of creating the changes you seek.

DAVID: I'd like to not have to initiate every time. I'd like for her to want me sometimes too. I'd like for her to put in more effort. Even just wearing sexy underwear . . . just something to show me she was thinking about it.

GINO: What I really want is intimacy. I go to these Grindr hookups because I feel expected to. It's part of gay culture to be out fucking all the time. I actually don't like it. But no one knows that. I look like the biggest whore around, but actually, I'd like a boyfriend.

CYNTHIA: I want him to go down on me. I love it.

CAROLYN: I'd like to experience group sex. I think it would be amazing.

FIONA: I'd just like to have an orgasm.

DARREN: I want to feel connected during sex. I don't want to just feel like a piece of meat. She just gets on top of me and grinds her way to orgasm. I want more intimacy. I want her to touch me more.

SUNU: I'd like to not worry about my erection going down or coming too soon. I'd like to feel sexually confident, that I can please him.

LISA: I want for us to be more adventurous. I want to fuck outdoors. I want to have a threesome with another woman. I want him to watch me fuck other men. I want to watch him be fucked by a man.

Risk, Consent, and You

> A ship is always safe at the shore—but that is not what it is built for.

—Albert Einstein

Our bodies and erotic imaginations are not designed to be solely vehicles for thought. When our thoughts remain locked away in the safety of our minds, we extinguish any opportunity for flames of passion to ignite. Our privacy offers us retreat and safety should we need it. We are not compelled to disclose anything and everything to another. Simply getting used to trusting ourselves with that information is vital. Allowing ourselves to experience it forms the foundation of getting our sea legs with risk-taking.

In the previous chapter, we looked at the Wheel of Consent as a model for understanding the dynamics of touch. Anything that happens outside the circle can be experienced or interpreted as a violation of consent. Consent is a complex and tricky thing, and much more nuanced than simply "yes" or "no." It requires inquiry into our conditions for good sex (chapter 6) what we want, what we don't want, and what we might consider asking for if we feel brave enough to take the risk.

Consent is not simply something that happens on first dates. It is something we must engage with regularly in any and all of our sexual encounters, whether we are in long-term relationships or having a string of one-night stands. Because consent is a constant process, it's essential that managing it respectfully becomes a cornerstone of all your sexual adventures, no matter what your level of interest or experience is. In order to thrive sexually, consent is not optional, it's essential.

An alternative model to the Wheel of Consent, though not nearly as thorough, has been developed by Planned Parenthood. In true all-American style, they have adopted the acronym of FRIES to provide a memorable framework of what consent can look like.

- *Freely given.* Doing something sexual with someone is a decision that should be made without pressure, force, manipulation, or while drunk or high.
- *Reversible.* Anyone can change their mind about what they want to do, at any time. Even if you've done it before or are in the middle of doing it, you can stop, change or take a break without needing to justify it. We don't need to justify a "yes" and, for the same reasons, we needn't justify a "no."
- *Informed.* Be honest. If you do not want a certain place touched, for example, "I do not want any anal anything today" (even though you did it last week and it was fantastic), and your partner disregards that—that is not consent.
- *Enthusiastic.* If someone isn't excited, or really into it, that's not consent. While Planned Parenthood intend this model for teens and younger adults, possibly with little sexual experience, the idea of "enthusiasm," while well-intentioned, can put a damper on risk-taking. Instead, I prefer *Engaged.* "Engaged" means we are agreeing to something (similar to the "allowing" quadrant and the "willingness" anchor in the Triangle of Satisfaction) but with a degree of trepidation, which is made explicit. Our *conditions* are firmly expressed and in place and our capacity to reverse or revoke the decision is vital, without justification or fuss. We are not merely being dragged along, but actively choosing to do something, despite it being a bet both ways.
- *Specific.* Saying yes to one thing (like using a sex toy together) doesn't mean they've said yes to using all sex toys or using sex toys every time you have sex.

Distinguishing Types of Risk

Enthusiasm around risk-taking is a complex frontier. On one hand, we know we need to do something differently in order to initiate the changes we seek but, on the other, the electric fence can be powerful. Sexual trauma expert Staci Haines says it's totally possible to feel desire and shame at the same time.[5]

We can often feel both fear and excitement in the same places in our bodies. For a lot of us, it's the belly. For others, it's the throat and chest. Because fear and excitement can feel similar physiologically, sometimes the distinction between what I call a "playful risk" and a "dangerous risk" can be hard to make.

A playful risk is something that feels expansive and is accompanied by a sense of "bigness." It feels like we are being drawn toward it, despite any discomfort. If we were to do it, it could be an invigorating experience.

In contrast, a dangerous risk makes us feel small. A dangerous risk seizes us up. A dangerous risk feels restrictive, oppressive, makes us jump back a little (or a lot). We retreat, feel small, or even feel sick. Both types of risk (we will explore risk more in the chapter on blockages) may increase our heart rate or cause a sweat, but a dangerous risk feels prohibitive while a playful risk offers incentive.

To help you reflect on your relationship with risk, the following prompts invite you to begin exploring how *you* have used risk-taking in other areas of your life to consider how it might apply in sex and rekindling desire. Some people are more inclined to be risk-averse, which is perfectly OK. If you know you are risk-averse, or you are finding the thought of doing this challenging, take a break. Don't charge on through.

What is your body telling you right now? Does it feel expansive or like it wants to jump back . . . or something else? Honor that. Practicing listening to your body is essential when practising risk-taking.

Take a moment to take three big, deep, full breaths. Focus on your exhale. This helps to activate your parasympathetic nervous system, which governs relaxation and stress management.

These prompts are designed to help you see how risk operates in your life. For some of you, even reading this chapter is a practice in risk-taking, and we are almost at the end. Well done! I commend you!

Activity: Understanding Risk

- When was the last time you took a risk (non-sexual) and it paid off? What was the context and how did it feel?
- Take yourself back to that time. Recall the circumstances surrounding that risk. What was helpful? What was not?
- How did you feel before you decided to take action?
- Where did you feel it? Can you describe the physical sensation?
- Was the feeling like anything else (e.g., excitement, anticipation, ecstatic, threatened)? Try to describe it here.

Sometimes fear and excitement can feel similar and we can find it difficult to distinguish between playful and dangerous risks. Try to recall one example of each from your life. They needn't be sexual.

- What was the playful risk?
- How did it feel emotionally?
- Where did you feel it physically? Can you describe it?
- How did you decide to take the risk? How did you take your foot off the brake?
- What did you gain (e.g., pleasure, fun, experience) or what became possible after that?
- What did you lose or what was shut down after that (e.g., critical self-talk)?
- What became clearer once your foot was off the brake or you were outside the electric fence?

Important: for the next question, *do not choose or focus on a traumatic memory* for this activity, especially if you do not have access to ongoing support. Be mindful of your own limitations and *only* choose something that is not triggering for you. Alternatively, leave this part of the activity if it feels too confronting.

- What was the dangerous risk you said no to, or wish you had said no to?
- How did it feel emotionally?
- Where did you feel it physically? Can you describe it?

- How did you decide to take the risk?
- What did you gain or what would you have liked to have gained (e.g., practice in saying no, avoiding losing money, speaking your mind)?
- What did you lose or what was minimized or what would you have liked to have lost or minimized (e.g., anxiety, shame, fear)?

Finally, try this activity again, but this time consider a rewarding or playful sexual risk that you took. It needn't be dramatic but simply something of significance to you.

- What was the playful sexual risk?
- How did it feel emotionally?
- Where did you feel it physically? Can you describe it?
- How did you decide to take the risk?
- What did you gain, or what became possible after the risk was taken (e.g., pleasure, fun, experience)?
- What did you lose or what was shut down or quietened after the risk was taken (e.g., shame, fear, anxiety, being distracted, disconnection from partner, body numbness)?

Turning Ideas into Action
In the "Time for Reflection" in this chapter, we got curious. Go back to your notes for that section and look at what you wrote. Taking inspiration from there, consider:

- What erotic activity would encompass how you want to feel? (or)
- What you would like to try? (and)
- What would you want your partner to magically know about it?

Allow whatever comes to mind to be there. Try not to shut it down. If nothing comes at all, do not worry. It could be that you need more time to get comfortable with this idea. It could be that your brakes network is working overtime to protect you.

Stick with it. This is part of the process of risk-taking. Once you have something, allow yourself to really feel it viscerally.

If you are a visual person, imagine it. See yourself doing it. Notice how it feels. Notice the feelings that rise in your throat, chest, and belly. Notice if there is an urge to shut it down. Notice that urge, but instead of acting on it, allow it to be there and stick with the fantasy. Breathe.

If you are not visually oriented, feel yourself doing the activity. Feel yourself "feeling" how you *want* to feel. Notice the sensations that accompany it. If they are uncomfortable or unpleasant, that's OK. Simply breathe gently, focus on your exhale, and wait for the discomfort to pass. Once it passes, return to the fantasy of feeling how you long to feel.

If visualizing or feeling aren't your thing, try listening. Hear yourself doing the activity. Hear the environment around you. Will music help you get in the mood? If so, what song? Go ahead and put it on.

You wrote it before . . . do you need to write more? Will words take you there? If so, go for it. Write it in its most descriptive detail.

Regardless of your process at this stage, the main thing is allowing yourself to commit to it. Remember this is just a fantasy. You aren't required to disclose it to *anyone*, except yourself.

- Imagine yourself doing the "thing."
- Imagine yourself feeling how you want to feel.
- Imagine yourself being understood by your partner, feeling safe enough to play freely, and managing any trepidation that arises.

By paying attention to your intention, you keep yourself moving and not stranded at the bus stop.

This may have felt like an edgy chapter for some and I commend you for sticking with it. Well done. Learning to feel your feelings, take risks, and challenge old patterns is part of breaking out of our old habits and creating a sex life that's as interesting as it is fun and fulfilling. But this can only happen on your terms, with your pleasure and boundaries firmly embedded in your explorations.

In the next chapter we'll take a look at the role of erotic fantasy as a tool of self-inquiry as well as being fodder for risk-taking and desire. We'll examine some common fantasies as well as old beliefs about the usefulness of sharing fantasies with a partner before deciding if it's a good thing for you to do in your relationship.

CHAPTER 11

~

The Erotic Imagination

Eroticism is, above all else, exclusively human: it is sexuality socialized and transfigured by the imagination and the will of human beings. The first thing that distinguishes eroticism from sexuality is the infinite variety of forms in which it manifests itself. Eroticism is invention, constant variation. Sex is always the same.

—Octavio Paz

In the realm of desire, many people immediately leap to sexual fantasies for inspiration. Their meaning, their enactment, and sometimes even the effect of recruiting fantasies into relationships to inspire a lackluster sex life. To this point, we have explored many of the elements of sex that create nourishing and satisfying sex lives, from the clinical to the esoteric. We've considered the physical and emotional components of sex along with our values and beliefs. In this final section, we bring the imagination and meaning-making into play, to offer us a final element to the erotic template before we consider how to communicate this to those who need to know what we have uncovered about our desires.

How we distinguish fulfilling sex from mediocre sex is based on our ability and willingness to be engaged with ourselves in the moment.

Practical tools give us the confidence we need to move forward and bring our intentions and desires to life. But, for many, fulfilment of the body and emotions alone, is not enough. Going through the motions can feel just like another routine, another job, another thing on the to-do list. For such people, sex without the playful, creative, imaginative element will simply not entice them to play, nor sustain their attention. The vast mental landscapes that bring formation to creativity and playfulness provide one of the most powerful aphrodisiacs known to humanity: the erotic imagination.

Eroticism is the place where sex, lust, life, and its day-to-day shortcomings meet with playfulness, vitality, expression, and suppression. In our essence, as babies, we are sexual beings, but we are not *erotic* beings. Eroticism develops with time as we receive messages from those around us—including but not limited to caregivers, peers, and communities—about the world and how we are within it, combined with our responses to touch, visual, and emotional stimulation and care-taking. In other words, what we like is in constant formation, in response to our environment and how we interpret and experience it physically, mentally, emotionally, and even spiritually. Over time, the unique combination of expression, repression, stimulation, gratification, and growth form pathways within us that produce the essence of what we respond to at a sexual-psychological level. In effect, sex may be a collection of urges and acts, but eroticism is the way we make such practices and psychological exchanges *meaningful*. Embracing the paradoxes and complexities of our sexuality sits at the core of exploring our eroticism as adults.

Erotic fantasies are as common as daydreaming. The difference is that daydreams are not stigmatized in the way erotic fantasies are. The source of our fantasies, day dreams, and subsequent desire and arousal is always ourselves. The images, symbols, emotions, and activities are drawn from deep within us and are compelling enough to engage our imagination, for better or worse. Other people, objects, scenarios, or beings may invoke or inspire it, but, ultimately, it's *us* that turns us on. Whether physical, mental, or emotional—we must give ourselves over to the experience to *feel* it all.

Yet our erotic fantasies are not always of an explicitly "sexual" nature. By definition, *sexual* fantasies are likely to involve sex of some kind, which many of us tend to associate with "pants-off" activities.

Touching our own or someone else's genitals with hands, mouths, other genitals, or objects in this context is this definition of a sexual fantasy. However, as sex therapist David Ortmann suggests in his book *Sexual Outsiders*[1](coauthored with Richard Sprott, PhD), *erotic* fantasies may or may not involve engagement with eroticism that moves beyond sex in more conventional contexts. Erotic fantasies may involve excitement about practices in which no clothing is removed at all, and the emphasis is on feelings, thoughts, or behaviors that engage our arousal beyond traditional genital sex practices. Such fantasies are experienced as exciting and arousing, and are therefore equally as valuable as *sexual* fantasies. The wonder of exploring the edges in this way also means such narratives may offer insight into how to access a lagging libido when excitement and stimulation can be found through less conventional erotic practices.

Imagining ourselves in a hot tryst with a (several) flight attendant(s), being desired by strangers at a sex party, doing unspeakable things with a celebrity crush, being punished by a cruel mistress, or getting paid for sexual acts we'd never do in real life are among some of the common sexual fantasies people describe when allowed to explore them freely. For others simply being validated by a sexy stranger or offered emotional refuge from the daily grind by way of a sensual massage is enough to help us engage with eroticism in a way that allows joy without burden. For many of us, our fantasies are the one aspect of our lives we have total control over, so whether we are the protagonist or the recipient—we are in control of what happens and how; thus, they provide the perfect soothing balm or exciting distraction to life's daily ups and downs. Psychologist Michael Bader even suggests that a good fantasy offers the problem and states the solution.[2] Fantasy is there to offer us insight into what makes us tick, whether we like it or not.

Fantasies are not intended to devalue the more mundane, repetitive, or even familiar aspects of sex but, rather, offer a portal into the erotic imagination that we can call on to kick-start lagging or blocked desire. Sexual / erotic fantasies needn't be elaborate or extensive. They can be a brief encounter or a longing for a specific act, object, or interpersonal dynamic. They can come in the form of images, sounds, emotions, or sensations, but what makes them compelling is that they arouse our senses and demand our attention.

Case Study: John

John was a young, gay man with a very common contemporary problem: unwanted erotic thoughts during sex. When I met John, he had been dating his current partner for six months and was feeling very connected and into the relationship. The sex was fulfilling, they communicated well—from the outside the prognosis was great!

Internally though, John battled with himself every time they had sex because he struggled to keep his mind on the job. The more aroused he got, the more his mind would wander to images from his previous sexual encounters, or images and clips he'd seen in porn. Racked with guilt and shame, John came to see me because the intrusive images had become too overpowering for him to bear. He was convinced these fantasies meant he didn't love his partner and he couldn't understand how he could be so in love and simultaneously be so desiring of others right in the middle of fucking the man he loved! He started doubting the relationship. His partner. And himself. He was convinced the images were some kind of sign or crucial information that he was heading in the wrong direction.

"How do you know these images mean you don't love your partner?" I asked. I was curious if he knew that people's minds wandered all the time—during sex, while driving, while waiting at the bank. They think about groceries, social media, domestic chores, that thing Sharon said on What's App, and, yes, memories of previous encounters or images from porn often pop into our heads when we least want them to.

"I don't know," he replied.

"If you momentarily thought about paying your bills or getting your car fixed during sex, would it make you think you wanted to have sex with your car?" I wondered.

"Of course not, that's ridiculous. A car is an inanimate object and these images are real people!" he retorted defiantly.

"You're correct," I said. "But my point is that these people, some of whom are long gone from your life and some of whom you've never met, are about as relevant to you now as a car, but because they are people not objects, you experience the very same intrusive thoughts differently. If it were a car or a bill you could dismiss it, but when it's people, it has meaning."

"That's right," he said. "That's it, it's what it means!"

I continued, "and yet we are no more certain of the meaning of erotic images during sex than we are of the meaning of bills and cars during sex, except for the weight we apply to them."

He paused and considered.

"But afterward, I feel really bad." He went on, "I feel like I've cheated. Like I abandoned him for these other people, people I know I don't care about. That's what makes it really hard."

"I see," I said. "At the time it feels OK, but during the aftermath, your mind, the very same one that throws the images to you, also decides to make meaning of the images, and decides you must be the bad guy. And you *believe* it! That sounds rough!" I concluded.

"It is. It's really hard." He welled up and let two small tears drip down his cheeks.

As we dug in further, we realized what was also being challenged by the images were his values around strength, loyalty, and monogamy. In his head, his inner critic declared he was actually cheating on his partner every time they had sex. John was a prisoner of his own erotic imagination and it was destroying his peace of mind.

As we explored John's values of loyalty and monogamy, I wondered how he fared showing loyalty *toward himself*. During sex, the erotic thoughts came and went, and in the moment, he enjoyed them. But afterward, he lost touch with the loyalty he cherished so much at other times.

He knew this was unsustainable and I explained to him that there was no therapeutic technique on Earth that could stop him from having the thoughts he had. But the good news was we could work on how he *responded* to the thoughts by focusing on the very things he valued most: strength and loyalty.

"What would you do if this was happening to a buddy of yours?" I asked. "If you saw your best friend being verbally abused, the way your mind berates you, by someone at the gym—would you just walk off and abandon him or would you do something to comfort him?"

"Of course I'd take care of him. I'm loyal." He looked me right in the eye.

The lights slowly started to come on. John realized he wasn't offering himself the same level of loyalty and kindness he would offer another who was struggling with being abused. He was abandoning his values of strength and loyalty by berating himself over the lusty thoughts he couldn't control.

"What about," I asked, "if instead of looking for a universal meaning behind these images, that applied to all of us, there was room for you to inquire about the feelings these images evoke for you, personally. What would that open up for you?"

He thought hard about this. It hadn't occurred to him that he could interpret these images any way he wanted. He defaulted to a narrative of shame because the collective understanding in our culture is, when you're in love, really truly in love, you only have eyes for that one person, or certainly only one at a time. Because of this cultural association, John had fused with the idea that his thoughts were shameful. That he must be a bad person and that the most likely interpretation was that he mustn't really love or desire his partner if he had to add spice to their sex by thinking about others.

"You mentioned that during sex you enjoy the images. What do you enjoy? What do they offer you?" I inquired.

"Well," he began, "It makes sex hotter and I enjoy myself more. The more turned on I am the more I want my partner. . . ." He looked confused, "So I guess that's a good thing?" he whispered to himself, softening his gaze.

"Sure," I agreed. "It certainly *could* be a good thing, especially if it helps you enjoy yourself more and want your partner more too."

Initially, John struggled to accept that these thoughts were not actually a *part* of him, but something he was experiencing as a temporary state that he had little control over. Shame has an unmistakable way of making us feel we are so deeply flawed that nothing can shift the weight of our burden, not even our most cherished values. Culturally he, like all of us, had believed that love and desire were the same (even though his life experiences were very much to the contrary), and if we were to *ever* think of another during sex, it must mean *only* negative repercussions. Even if the images offered him more of what he wanted at the time—pleasure and connection—shame convinces us we are bad for indulging in the thoughts in the first place, even if we cannot help it. He was abandoning his values of strength and loyalty by berating himself over the lusty thoughts he couldn't control. When he realized that the very things he valued most, he wasn't offering to himself, he was able to change the story in his head about sex and allow himself to be kinder to himself after sex, which actually brought him closer to his partner. By expanding the way he embodied his values, he was able to create room for his eroticism, his discomfort and his values all at the same time. The bonus was that, over time, he became more relaxed. And as he was being kinder to himself, the erotic thoughts became less intrusive, and he was more able to focus on staying present during and after sex.

As we recall from the brain science of chapter 5, we are only just beginning to understand the relationship between the brain and sex, and we are even less knowledgeable about the relationship between the mind and sex. But what we do know is that intrusive thoughts of all types happen in many contexts to everyone, all the time, and are something we all have to learn to live with and manage—whether during a meeting at work or in the middle of sex with someone we really like. We also learned that what we desire, what we like, and what we want can be different. Like ice cream on a hot or cold day, when the context changes, our desire changes. But shame around consuming cold food on hot days is less overwhelming for many of us than enjoying erotic imagery designed to induce pleasure. For us, the struggle is making peace with our experience of the erotic imagination before condemning it to destruction.

Lust versus Disgust

Fantasy and eroticism have traditionally been difficult to study and define. Their nature is subjective and inherently idiosyncratic, so what is "hot" for one may be "disgusting" for another. Studies have suggested that disgust is an "adaptive" or learned psychological response to something outside of ourselves that compels us to move away from the object of our repulsion. In contrast, lust is also an adaptive response that compels us to move toward the object we find appealing. In an erotic context however, some may find opposition between these two experiences in the form of considering a series of sexual acts that mentally we find triggering, repulsive, or disgusting, yet when sexually turned on and aroused, transform almost like magic from "disgust" to "lust."

The cognitive links between "lust" and "disgust" have been shown to interact powerfully, yet counter-productively, within our brains and bodies when it comes to sex, sometimes, but studies (of women) have also revealed some surprising evidence about how disgust may also be transformed.[3] In a control group of women invited to participate in a series of "disgusting" sexual and non-sexual acts, researchers Charmaine Borge and Peter J. de Jong found that women asked to perform such acts (e.g., eating a cookie placed next to a worm on a plate, or sipping from a cup with a large [fake] insect in it) described significantly less disgust when they were sexually aroused than when they were not. The study hypothesized that the presence of physical sexual arousal produced an effect within the body and mind that can override the "disgust" mechanism. This may explain how some of the most common "disgust" elicitors; open mouth kissing, sweat, oral sex juices, rimming (licking the anal opening), and bad body odor can be revolting in one moment and intoxicating in another. The trick is, for those for whom the space between those two places feels daunting, finding the motivation to get to the other side requires more than just will power but actually involving the body in such a way as to produce *arousal*. This suggests that if full sexual arousal is present first, the disgust factor may be significantly reduced. This is great news for lovers whose erotic longings may appear to be mismatched, although similar studies have not been conducted in men or other genders to date. That said, anecdotally, my therapeutic experience has suggested that, while some differences between men and women indeed appear to exist, there are more similarities than distinctions, which allow us to paint more broadly when looking at arousal, lust, and disgust in all people on the gender spectrum.

Fantasy versus Reality
When we daydream about fantasy holidays, ultimate jobs or travel adventures we allow ourselves full permission to experience the fantasy. Such flights-of-fancy are not scrutinized by the same moral policing that our sexuality is. But the truth is, while in many cases we may actually want to travel, have a dream job, or spend a week on a yacht eating caviar—we may not actually *want* to do the things we fantasize about sexually / erotically. Instead, these fantasies can offer a gateway into aspects of our emotions that we are trying to reconcile in our day-to-day lives. I often describe these confusing experiences as part of the

"sex bucket"—like a bucket full of fish heads and fish guts before being turned into nutritious stock. The "sex bucket" is the place difficult and incomplete emotions go to get processed when they feel too difficult to deal with. In other words, complex erotic fantasies can often be the residents of the emotional "too hard" basket.

Historically, sexual fantasies were often misunderstood and thought to exist only in the minds of so-called deviants and perverts. While "deviants" and "perverts" certainly have sexual fantasies, so too does everyone else, including asexuals—although in lower numbers and potentially more fulfilling at the erotic imagination end of the spectrum, rather than the physically embodied end.[4] While sexual / erotic fantasies are extremely common and something many are at peace with, they can sometimes present as troubling, especially when they offer an experience of ourselves that sits in contrast with who we *think* we are.

For example, if we value monogamy and are in a monogamous relationship, it may be difficult to reconcile a recurring sexual fantasy about someone other than our partner. The presence of this other person in our erotic mental landscape may be experienced as cheating by our own personal morals, and lead to feelings of shame and guilt, thus making the fantasy difficult to engage with let alone share. When this happens, we may feel an urgent need to remove the fantasy because what we *think* of the fantasy (our ideals, beliefs, and personal values) and how we *feel* about it (turned on, excited, and aroused) may be in opposition (like we explored in chapter 6), and can become a source of discomfort, shame, dissociation, and detachment. Another way we may experience this is that it's not at all uncommon for men identifying as strictly heterosexual to find themselves fantasizing about erotic exchanges with other men, or dressing in "women's" underwear, or watching their wives or girlfriends having sex with other men, and being turned on by the presence of another man's body. While the "normalness" of such fantasies is established insofar as it's not uncommon[5] the person who has the fantasies may be worried about what that "says" about them. Does it mean they are gay? Transgender? Bisexual? Or something else entirely? Perhaps. Perhaps not. In searching for meaning based on fantasies alone, we omit the context in which the fantasies happen (remember, it's all about the Self) and how we see

Time for Reflection

What are some of the beliefs you inherited from your community and culture about sexual fantasies and the people who have them? What about people who act on them? What impact has that had on your relationship with having fantasies and enjoying them? Have you ever experienced intrusive sexual thoughts, like John, that you interpreted as shameful, even if you experienced pleasure from them at the time? If so, how did you reconcile the two or how could you begin to think of them in a kinder, gentler way, to be more curious (like the Triangle of Satisfaction) of what they bring you before deciding you're definitely a bad person?

ourselves and our "real" lives. In such contexts, the fantasizer may not want to act on these things at all, yet they offer comfort momentarily at the end of a long day, as masturbation fodder before sleep, or an escape from the spreadsheets that need attending to before noon tomorrow. The only *trouble* with this is solely upon what we *interpret* this to mean—and how much value we place upon it.

What Kinds of Things Do People Fantasize About? And Why?

The short answer is, the sky's the limit. Any searches for porn these days reveal a multitude of erotic fantasies. Researcher Justin Lehmiller's studies reveal that it may also work the other way around, insofar as porn can influence our fantasies. [6] What we like to watch or, perhaps, are drawn to watch (wanting and liking are different, as we discovered earlier in chapter 5) and what we like to *do*, however, can be really different Nor does it say anything to us about what these fantasies mean, if in fact there is any meaning at all.

Traditionally, mental health communities have been especially responsible for the unnecessary pathologizing of erotic fantasies and sex. We can trace this back to Freud, whose insistence that "happy people don't fantasize" started a trend toward such ignorance. Moreover, the overwhelming influence of Western romanticism, insisting that love and sex are the same, has had its way meddling in erotic freedom. Popular opinion would have us believe that any fantasy that exists outside a romance context "must" be problematic and a sign of being "unhealthy." This isn't true. That said, fantasies can offer us a portal into what engages us, without the need to pathologize, change, or shame what arouses us.

Fantasies can speak to parts of ourselves that we place out-of-mind in order to get on with our lives. The blips and bumps in the road, the hits to our self-esteem, or the places that our emotions can take us, all have an effect on even the most stoic among us.

Perhaps, fantasies about sex with strangers may be speaking to a desire to be free of pressure, duty, and responsibility to others in our day-to-day lives. Being with strangers in this scenario allows us the space to be free of responsibilities and emotional obligations. After all, with strangers, there is no need for discussion or negotiations. They know exactly what you want and are willing to please. Ultimately, it's all about you. Fantasies about a person we actively dislike—a boss, an ex, or a teenage nemesis—may be a way of coming to terms with the dynamic between us, taking control of the situation in our minds to make peace with it in the real world. Often times, such fantasies are about what that person *represents*—rather than who they *are*. Likewise, fantasies about being with a heartthrob type may speak to a longing for perfection or acceptance that feels out of reach in our real-world life. Not all fantasies involve "the Erotic Equation," but many will involve elements that sit in contrast with how we see ourselves.

One of the most common fantasies I have encountered working with women are rape fantasies and fantasies of being overpowered. In 100 percent of such cases I have encountered clinically, *none* of the women said they wanted for this to happen, *ever*, in real life. But there is something about the role of power in (women's) fantasies that is one of the most intoxicating aphrodisiacs of all. This helps explain why bodice rippers like everything from Mills and Boon to *Fifty Shades* share a theme of a strong figure taking control through force. While the quality of such narratives is certainly up for debate, the fact remains, the themes are pervasive and reflected in my therapy room as well as bookstore shelves and porn sites globally. And this is not solely in the realm of women. Men too can enjoy the fantasy of being sexually subordinate without necessarily wanting to do anything about it. The Crash Pad

Series referenced in chapter 10 centers queer and non-binary bodies, and self-scripted and self-directed stories, many of which depict scenarios involving overcoming ambivalence with power.

Fantasies involving power play may be speaking to a desire to gain or relinquish control regarding our private lives, work lives, or roles in society. Fantasising about power dynamics from consensual to non-consensual are some of the most popular erotic fantasies because power dynamics in these contexts can create such sensorial arousal. And while fantasies about power are among the most common, they too are often linked to fantasies about gender, which, in most cultures, have ties that bind. Fantasies about gender may be about a longing to break free of the social obligations placed upon us by gendered restrictions, while fantasies of being the center of attention and desired by large groups of people may be about a longing to be seen and valued as a person of worth or importance, or part of something much larger than the individual self. Likewise, fantasies of shame and humiliation may allow for acceptance of parts of the Self that have been socially rejected, thus placing the fantasizer in agreement with the judgment and allowing a place for pain to be accepted and integrated in a meaningful way. Fantasies about or involving objects or locations may provide an opportunity to externalize certain feelings unrelated to sex, so we can get to know them better from a manageable distance. And sometimes fantasies are just exactly what they are—excitement about being with, wearing, or doing certain things simply because we enjoy them with no hidden meaning or ulterior motive. They're just good old-fashioned fun. They may be carnal and deeply sexual, or may be romantic and very emotionally oriented. After all, we like what we like, and as long as no one is being (non-consensually) hurt—enjoy!

Peak Erotic Experiences

Navigating the space between lust and disgust takes inquiry, and one tool that can lead us to understand more about how those places operate within us is our own erotic history and imaginings. Eroticism exists in the mind, the imagination, in lived experience, and in the visceral "memories" of the physical body. The practice of diving deep into these memorable erotic experiences allows us to focus on the details that most stand out to us in our recollections—physically, emotionally, energetically, and mentally. This intoxicating blend of information is the essence of what Jack Morin, PhD, defined as the "peak erotic experience."[7] Morin's unique "Sexual Excitement Survey" (not to be confused the Dual Control Model's sexual excitement scale [SES]), conducted in the 1980s and 1990s, invited hundreds of men and women (straight, lesbian / gay, and bisexual) to describe, in detail, their hottest and most memorable erotic experiences. Morin posited that such memories and visceral reflections can tell us a lot about what drives our emotional desires and longings, and by making such information accessible in conscious and attentive ways, we can actually allow our minds to lead us to the path of greatest possible erotic growth and exploration.

Discover Your Peak Erotic Experiences
The unique blend of who we are, what we believe, how we feel, and our sexual experiences to date, combined with our capacity to imagine, form the foundation of what Morin calls the "Core Erotic Theme" (CET)[8]. The CET allows us to identify the stories—the narratives, the fantasies, or the experiences—that most ignite our erotic imagination. One way that he suggests we do this is to reflect on some of our most memorable fantasies or intimate encounters. Sex may or may not be involved in these because peak eroticism isn't necessarily connected to sex in the conventional ways we imagine it—that is, involving genitals, penetration, and so forth.

Start by taking in three deep, full breaths. Focus on your exhale to give your body permission to relax. Allow yourself to float mentally / imaginatively through time, recalling some of your favorite erotic experiences from real life or from your private fantasies. Have a notebook or device ready to write, draw, or in some way record the information from the following activity. Choose a fantasy that has some resonance for you.

What fantasy is most likely to get you aroused? Allow yourself to really move toward it with everything in your being—mental, physical, and emotional.

Reflect on the fantasy and consider what stands out about it the most. The emotions, the imagination, the creative freedom to go places and really *feel*. Record the answers to the following prompts as a guide for working with your fantasies.

1. What makes / made the fantasy so exciting?
2. What conditions enabled it to get played out?
3. Who does it involve? (It's not necessarily about *them*, remember?)
4. What is it about the other people involved that arouses / excites / engages you?
5. What are they doing?
6. What attributes do *they* embody that engage you?
7. What attributes do *you* embody that engage you? (Many people imagine their body / personality to be different to how it is in real life.)
8. What is the most intense point of the fantasy?
9. What do *you* think makes this so exciting for you?

Perhaps your fantasy involved entirely visual elements, power play elements, taboo elements, or with no clothing removed at all? Perhaps it's more romantically oriented with a very strong emotional connection between you and the other(s) involved. Allow yourself to go with whatever comes up. Something; anything at all, even if it doesn't make sense. Even if you don't have fantasies in the traditional sense; maybe fragmented erotic thoughts—grab onto them too. Clothing, a look, a feeling of being alive, desired, shunned, devious, naughty, wanted, important, ashamed, submissive, powerful, in control, overpowered . . . the list is endless. There is some juicy and useful information in there that made part of you come alive, even if it stands at cross purposes of what we *think* we're supposed to feel or experience when it comes to our sexuality.

This is a gateway to your eroticism and your *Core Erotic Theme.*

If you can, repeat the exercise for another fantasy. Even several more.

Look out for patterns or similarities that occur across fantasies or experiences. Morin notes fantasies have several themes:

- Firsts and surprises. (Not the *first* of the first but, rather, the *first* orgasm, *first* squirt, *first* with a new situation)
- Idyllic situations or partners. (E.g., the beach, a bathroom at a party, rose petals, a dirty laneway, a perfectly equipped dungeon, a lush forest, under the sea, a *tidy* bedroom, having a perfect body,

having larger / smaller body parts than in real life, being another gender, etc.)

- Extensions or restrictions of time. (People will describe a loss of time, a feeling of otherworldliness, hours passing. Or the *last* time; with a lover leaving or dying. A quickie in a closet or public space, immediacy or orgasm and bliss despite the time limitations.)

Consider what it is about these recurring moments that appeals to you?

Being able to identify and hopefully name these sensations or feelings is part of identifying the most powerful themes in your fantasy world.

If nothing obvious stands out to you, reflect on what was arousing or attractive about the situation. Recall the erotic equation: Attraction + Obstacles = Excitement.

Consider any things that got in your way, including yourself and your assessment of the situation. For example:

This is bad.
This is disgusting.
I'm a bad person for thinking this.
I wouldn't do this in any other circumstances.

It may seem counterintuitive, but feeling anxious, guilty, ashamed, humiliated, and even angry can inflame passionate sensations leading to erotic engagement. The standard couple's therapy trope of love and intimacy leading to great sex is simply not true for everyone every time, and if you are one of those people, you are not alone, nor are you damaged, weird, or broken. Erotic excitement can come from many sources. The tricky part, however, can be finding people to share these with and who are willing to engage in these with you, should you want to, as a discussion or for enactment.

Using Fantasies for Personal Development

While studies of our fantasies (across gender and orientation) and their meanings are inconclusive, it is understood that our sexual fantasies offer us a portal into areas of our lives that bring us meaning and excitement but not necessarily always pleasure. Sometimes, acting on the fantasy can be anti-climactic or can leave us feeling worse than the anxiety it initially created. Often what makes the fantasy powerful is the fact that it is just that—a fantasy! Its purpose is to help process emotions and complexities, but not necessarily a reflection of any latent erotic desire to act on. Any attempt to enact it, kills its allure immediately. On occasion, this part of the game can be a crushing blow for the fantasizer, as the one thing they have held dear and cherished as the greatest erotic (and therefore emotional) high, comes crashing down with nothing to replace it. Not all fantasies involve uncomfortable or controversial emotions, but many will include an aspect that does not fit comfortably inside our concept of who we are. It's easy to avoid by dismissing these fantasies as "wrong" or avoiding their existence entirely. The discomfort our fantasies reveal, offer an opportunity to explore what makes us retreat from our eroticism or from the eroticism of others, including our partners. When we are quick to judge, criticize ourselves or others, or withdraw from lovers because of fantasies, it may be useful to slow down and be attentive to that which is making us uncomfortable. It may also be helpful to consider what it is about your fantasy or your partner's fantasy that is threatening or unacceptable. Consider its effect on your own CET. Is there something about the fantasy that makes you see yourself or your partner differently? Collect all of these reflections in your notebook as it adds to your erotic template.

In these situations, it can be very easy to jump to conclusions about what a fantasy says about us without any evidence to confirm it. As if the presence of this *one* fantasy overrides all the other qualities we possess or embody, including being a good friend, parent, lover, spouse, member of the community, therapist, employee, or boss.

If anyone knew this about me, they'd dump me, for sure!

So instead, we abandon *ourselves*—vow to never engage with that part of ourselves, bury it deep, deep, way down. After a while, its presence becomes a distant memory but is still felt as a sense of

- numbing,
- dullness,

- bleakness or lethargy,
- a lack of enthusiasm for play, or
- a cloak of shame that keeps us away from connecting with ourselves.

For some it can even manifest as

- depression,
- loneliness, and, you guessed it,
- no libido.

As an alternative, try resisting the urge to believe the meaning you place on it as the absolute truth and, instead, practice considering it an opinion. Seek out or allow yourself to imagine several other opinions. Instead of certainty, adopt a little curiosity. Put your investigative journalist hat on and allow yourself to consider the fantasy from various points of view. What other meanings might be possible in a fantasy about claiming or relinquishing power, for example? Remember, curiosity from the Triangle of Satisfaction is an important element here. What contexts might make this more digestible for you? Try researching (Googling) the fantasy and see if you can get a sense of how popular it is. How common it is. Does it ease your mind to know others feel similarly to you? Lehmiller's research into popular fantasies offers us insight into the prevalence and breadth of erotic fantasies of Americans, data which helps us see ourselves in a much clearer and hopefully more compassionate light. The more we can practice seeing fantasies for what they are, normal aspects of human imagination, the more we can learn from them and even allow them to be our sign post on an otherwise lonely erotic path back to pleasure.

Should I Tell?

While old-school sex therapy often spoke of sharing fantasies with our partners as a means of connection and a definitive insight into the kinds of sex we want, contemporary approaches suggest it is neither necessary nor is it an accurate jumping off point for negotiating new activities, especially if your fantasies are out of sync with one another, or even within yourself. Sexual fantasies offer a space for us to play, learn, and grow, as well as an opportunity to process ourselves, which is not necessarily fun for you or your partner(s). Throwing your erotic inquiries or longings onto your partner without their consent can lead to burdens and miscommunications. So it's essential that you tread lightly, gently, and respectfully when unpacking the wondrous world of erotic fantasies. They are deeply personal and not to be judged or scrutinized with anything other than empathy and curiosity. One of the great things about fantasies is that they are yours and yours alone, only to be shared how, when, and if you want.

Fantasies can be complex terrain. Hopefully the information contained in this chapter will liberate you from some of the unnecessary stigma of fantasies and for others be the source of inspiration for hotter more meaningful sex. Regardless of how you integrate this information, I invite you to marvel at the mind's capacity to express itself. Using the content of your fantasies may or may not feel like the perfect tool for boosting your libido, personal healing, or cultivating self-awareness and personal growth. With willingness on your side, you may find extraordinary liberation and relief by following the trail of inquiry through your fantasies—sexual, romantic, or otherwise.

You're invited to be gentle and try to suspend judgment of yourself and others when navigating this information. Suspending judgment needn't mean compromising one's moral compass or personal values but, rather, encouraging compassion and exploration of complexity. For it can be *through* adversity that many of us experience the most growth, change, and liberation from the shackles that reduce and refrain us, sometimes creating a deadening of desire. It is generally not a fast process but one that can produce the answers to the erotic challenges we find most vexing. Only in a safe place do we feel most comfortable to reveal ourselves to ourselves and potentially to others. Such discoveries will not be feasible without the willingness to set aside critical assessments and be immersed in the presence of the truths revealed to the open-hearted.

And with compassion in mind, in the next chapter we begin to consider how to share this information we have gathered about ourselves and our erotic template with another. Where to start. How to say it. And what to expect. Take a breath and perhaps a break. I'll join you there.

CHAPTER 12

~

Talking about Sex Like It Matters

The day came when the risk to remain tight in a bud was more painful than the risk it took to blossom.

—Anaïs Nin

By now, you likely have come to recognize that sexual desire is far more individual, unique, and idiosyncratic than Disney, porn, and romance novels would have us believe. It's way more nuanced than any sex advice column could do justice to. It's not simply a case of eyes meeting across a crowded room and then staying blissfully entwined forever. It may start that way for some, but it never stays that way without effort. Keeping erotically connected in relationships takes energy and commitment. Throughout this book, you have been investigating, developing, and refining your erotic template. Discovering more of who you are. What you want. What you like. How you like it. Under what conditions you like it. Under what conditions you *don't* like it. Why you do it. What you can do internally when you need to change course. What makes something satisfying for you. What activates your brakes. What you need to unlearn and where you still have places to remain curious. All of this, my friend, is your erotic template. *All of it*. And it's always a work in progress. In this chapter we will start to bring it all together and help you learn to communicate and share this knowledge with the people around you who most need to know. A sometimes tricky endeavor, but one we can learn step-by-step.

Understanding and Sharing Your Sexual Values

There's no singular reason why partners experience sex problems. Sex problems are as varied as sexual motivations. The trouble is, as I am sure you now know, when we consider questions such as "why we have sex," we find that our motivations are different to those of our lovers. The importance we place on these values can shift with time too. Differences between partners are normal, so intimacy issues and difficulties in sexual communication will come up over and over again. Without a degree of sexual and emotional intelligence, partners can find themselves with limited resources to manage these complexities.

In chapter 6, we looked at what motivates us to have sex and under what conditions we most enjoy it.

Now you have the chance to consider how your motivations might become values, things you consider important, which influence what you want to gain, discover, or experience from sex each time you do it, or on very specific occasions. For example, there may be times you are more emotionally sensitive than others: What do you want to feel? Or, perhaps more physically charged than others, in terms of the Wheel of Consent Model (chapter 9): What do you want to offer or what gift do you want to receive? Perhaps you want to experiment with a new move, technique, practice. A new experience of power, surrender, dominance, or submission. Or you want some affirmation of your relationship, gender, attractiveness, power, desirability, and so on. Each time we have sex can be different than the previous, and having a format for communicating about these values helps us know where we are at, and where our partners are at, before we get into it.

Look at the list of values below. It can be helpful to think of them as items on a menu and you are assessing your appetite *today*. Your appetite isn't the same every single day, so we are looking at this case by case. Are there others not listed that are important to you? Perhaps now you have discovered some new ones you want to add, some you want to remove or some that are only true under certain conditions and circumstances. Circle the ones that pique your appetite today. Take as many as you like.

excitement
comfort
to feel wanted
as a favor
to feel attractive or desired
to keep the relationship
distraction from other things
boredom
exercise
for money /gifts / food
so you can be owed something
  back
to feel good in your body
obligation
help partner's mood
pity
to try something new
connection
intimacy
to feel powerful
because you're angry
because you don't want the other
  person to feel rejected
out of frustration
to learn more about yourself
for fun
to pass the time
guilt
physical pleasure
to act out your fantasies
to wake up
to experience new parts of yourself
for the afterglow

to relax
because its expected
validation
confidence
habit / familiarity
procrastination
for release of tension
to feel better about your skills
to affirm / reinforce your gender
  identity
to heal wounds from the past
to prove something
to get pregnant
to reassure the other person
to experiment
to help calm your nerves / mind
to cheer yourself up
to stop the other person from
  pressuring you
to feel "normal"
free time
because you like someone
to get it over with
to show off your talents and
  knowledge
to relieve stress
to help you sleep
release
physical satisfaction
pleasure
connection
intimacy
well-being
romance

excitement	power/control/ surrender
spiritual experience	involves genitals
enough time	orgasm
varied activities	personal growth
sumptuous surroundings	self-understanding
being naughty / taboo	experimentation and creativity
to feel "normal"	self-expression
ecstatic	anything else?

Next, open to a new page in your notebook and make three columns. Name them "Super Important," "Important," and "Not Very Important." Rank your chosen menu items in your notebook in the column where they most fit for *today*. For example, certain values may be more relevant during partnered sex than solo sex. Others may be more relevant with one partner and not another. Of course, we needn't do all this every single time we have sex, but we can, should we want to. Doing this with a partner can help you know where you both are at and perhaps help you decide what activities you will do today and how to get the most pleasure from them according to your appetite.

Map Your Erotic Values
Another way to use this information is to plot the above information into a chart such as the one shown in figure 12.1. In this case, 0 means not at all important and 80 means extremely important. You can do this alone or with a partner to provide a visual representation of your erotic values and how you and your partner may be similar and different on that day. It's also helpful to use this chart as a point of discussion for exploring your motivations and expectations of sex, and also for tracking sexual satisfaction in a relationship over time.

Becoming fluent in personal and erotic values takes practice. They morph and change as we experience new emotions and sensations. They are the curveballs that bring purpose to our sexual exploration in passionate and challenging ways. When we are faced with dramatic change like illness or grief, sometimes sex is the place our difficult emotions go to get processed while we tend to other things. We withdraw, maybe we become uncharacteristically sexually charged, we develop an interest in something new, or we experience unexplained physical

Erotic Values

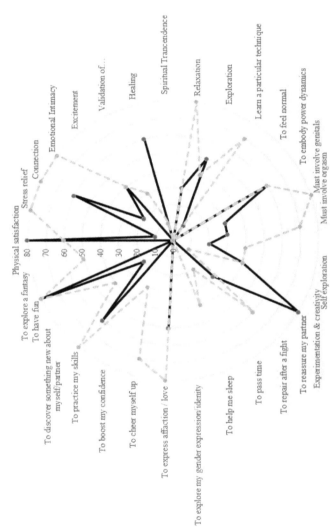

Figure 12.1. Erotic values.

pain. There are many ways emotional upheaval can manifest in our sexuality for better or for worse. It may not be "logical" but, for many of us, sex is the place where deep unresolved "stuff" goes to get addressed, in ways that other forms of logical analysis or emotional investigation cannot provide.

Case Study: Steve and Ed
"When we first got together, I really enjoyed sex with my husband, but over time it started to change a little. I didn't hate it, not at all, I just wanted it less often than him," Steve lamented in my office. "There were other ways of connecting that I got more from."

He continued, "But after he got sick, my enthusiasm really dropped off, but his didn't. During his illness, it became increasingly important to him that he have orgasms, because they became so difficult for him to have. Without them, sex became meaningless for him. In the past, orgasms were not an issue for him so he was less anxious about them. But the illness changed that. The sex we used to have was no longer possible and he became extremely frustrated. Nothing we tried seemed to help or change the way he felt and it was affecting our relationship."

Steve was terribly distressed by the entire situation. He was so grateful Ed had survived and yet so unable to tolerate his sexual anxiety much longer.

"If it had been up to me, I would have just given sex up completely at that time," Steve declared. "But he didn't want that at all. He would expect things of me that I found really challenging, because for him sex became very much about affirmation and gratification. This really changed the sexual dynamic between us for a while."

Steve's sexual motivations and values remained fairly constant throughout their upheaval. He knew sex for him was primarily about intimacy and connection. Both in their fifties, their erections had become steadily unreliable, but where his husband Ed was once motivated to make sex about joy and pleasure, it increasingly became about his need for validation—not of love, but health and power. Ed's erotic values had changed dramatically, but neither of them knew this at first. To be well enough to have sex meant he was still healthy, but to be well enough to orgasm meant he was still virile and potent; something he began to value increasingly as his health deteriorated. Orgasm to Ed meant he was still alive, and the desperation to remain on the planet became something only orgasm could validate.

Steve's frustration with his husband's orgasmic demands was pretty high by the time I met them. Steve was at his wit's end with him and Ed was struggling to manage the grief he was feeling around his ailing health. During recovery, he wasn't dying, but his connection to his sexuality felt like it was. It was changing. He was struggling and desperate. It took time for Ed to realize how his erotic values had changed and how the urgency he now experienced was taking its toll on Steve and their relationship. For Ed, orgasm was a matter of life and death, not of his body but his masculinity. He wasn't ready to be divorced from his sexuality, but his panic around the changes he was experiencing made him feel sex had become all or nothing. In his mind he was either a "man" or a "reject." He became stuck in an erotic bind and his values of "joy" and "pleasure" got usurped by his need to prioritize his virility over everything else. Without orgasms, Ed felt less of a man. This was new for both of them and was at the core of their crisis. It made sense that the relationship was strained and even more so now that their sex life was showing more than a few cracks.

Sexual Values and Communication
The truth is that some people continue with relationships where the sex has always been so-so, and feel quite content with that because, for them, the benefits of the relationship are not, nor ever have been, about sex. But others tolerate mediocre sex because they neither know how to discuss it nor even realize that they can. Unresolved feelings spill out into the bed, and unacknowledged values control sexual play, leaving partners feeling disconnected and disappointed. Being aware of which erotic values are controlling or motivating your relationship with sex makes it easier to understand and discuss. In the case of Steve and Ed, the challenges they were facing extended from the physical to the emotional as well. Ed's challenge was to practice allowing himself to feel vulnerable during intimacy instead of avoiding his more challenging emotions by insisting solely on repeated orgasmic release. By shifting his attention from his pain to his process, he learns that their vulnerability opens up a new level of awareness for him. It won't feel like it felt before, but if he is willing, he will feel something brand

new. Being emotionally "still," long enough to feel himself, was part of the challenge, and something Steve so desperately needed him to do. Slowing down enough to allow themselves to identify and accept the feelings they were experiencing was at the core of them managing the changes in their relationship and their sex life.

Choose Your Own Adventure

Recognizing that you have a choice when it comes to sexual intimacy can be a double-edged sword. For some, it marks a kind of liberation to create exactly the kind of relationship and sex life they would like, and for others, it activates fear and doubt because the rules of sex are not as clear-cut as they once were. Back in the day, sex was considered obligatory and functional. Discussions of sex and pleasure were taboo, so no one bothered. Sex was strictly heterosexual, whether you identified that way or not, and solely penis-in-vagina. Everyone knew the script and they stuck to it (or at least pretended to). These days we realize that for sex to be fulfilling and consensual, we have to talk about it. It's difficult to accept change at the best of times but when it's forced upon us through no one's fault, it can be a blow to the dynamic of a relationship. Changes in erotic values are usually a combination of many mixed and changing emotions. This is completely normal. The responsibility of freedom is great and this, too, applies to matters of the heart, the body, and eroticism.

Does *Your* Relationship Need to Be Sexual?

For many couples, sex is implicit in the nature of their relationship but rarely explicitly discussed. It is assumed that partners are also lovers, but it is merely an assumption. Couples often look at me dumbfounded when I ask the question: "Does this relationship need to be sexual?" It's usually something they have never considered, let alone ever been asked. But the truth is, some couples function perfectly well in sex-free relationships.

In some cases, they arrange to get their sex elsewhere or they go without quite willingly. For Steve, sex was simply not an essential part of the relationship and he was quite willing to give it up. For others, the sex comes and goes, and when it wanes a little, that is OK with them. Some are in actively "open relationships," where other emotional connections are allowed to flourish alongside sexual ones. Others, again, have an explicit and agreed "don't ask, don't tell" policy, meaning, it's understood that sexual connections happen outside the relationship, but they are not emotionally oriented and are not discussed in detail beyond logistics, if at all. Such couplings are not resentful but simply recognize the shortcomings of the relationship are such that sex needn't be on their agenda when they are excellent partners in so many other ways. The thinking is: "Why ruin a good thing with something like sex? After all, *sex in a relationship is not compulsory*—so why do it if you *really, really* don't want to?" Unless, of course, you do want it but you *really* want something different than what's being offered. Feeling challenged by such inquiry is completely normal, and this process often holds the answers to the solutions many of us seek when reconciling sex, eroticism, and relationships. In the next chapter we'll look more deeply into common blockages people experience on the path of desire.

What Does This Relationship Need?
Numerous studies into relationship satisfaction, including those by the Gottman Institute[1] have concluded that the key to effective relationships is kindness and generosity. This can be extended to sex as well. When couples cease being kind and generous to each other, relationships tend to suffer. Sometimes sex suffers as well. When freedom is restricted or demanded without consent, we enter the danger zone. Determining what we value when it comes to our partnerships more broadly than sex alone will determine how well we function in our intimate lives. Sex is not compulsory, but kindness and generosity are. When your desires don't match, it's not a quest to get anyone to change so dramatically that they feel so compromised they become resentful. Instead, the solution lies in your ability to communicate, listen, make allowances, understand, and accommodate each other and the relationship. In other words, it all comes down to your ability to engage the Triangle of Satisfaction to find solutions that are sustainable for both / all of you.

It can be helpful to see the relationship as a living entity too. Many times relationships are perceived as static, monolithic, unchanging, and self-perpetuating. But relationships are alive and in motion. They flourish or decay depending upon how we nourish them. Instead of thinking only about "what I need" or "what you need," it can be help-ful to consider the relationship like a child, a pet, or a plant—in need of nourishment from all involved to keep it alive on its own terms. Consider the relationship's needs as a third *living* entity.

It can be helpful to consider it like this: there's you, your partner, and then your relationship in the middle. That relationship has a life and needs of its own, yet it is connected to both of you and dependent upon both of you to nourish it. It may fall more to one side or another from time to time, but it requires care from both / all partners, just like a child might.

What Does a Sexual Relationship Need?
Understanding what your sexual relationship needs to nourish it can be daunting at the start, so it's helpful to consider what relationships need *in general.* Take a step back and think more broadly about relationships in general, instead of yours specifically at this stage. What kind of things do you think an intimate or personal relationship needs? There are no right or wrong answers. This is simply an opportunity to reflect on your ideas about what makes an intimate relationship work, or your ideal scenario. Consider other people's relationships that you admire. Who do you know that embodies these kinds of relational qualities? List the qualities in your notebook. Some suggestions are shown in figure 12.3. Add as many as you like.

Do this separately from your partner. When you are ready, come together to discuss your ideas. It can be helpful to draw the venn dia-gram shown in figure 12.2 and put shared ideas for "nourishment" into the "relationship" circle. Any that you don't agree on or are unsure about, you can place in your own circle as something you may seek out-side the relationship, or place outside the diagram for future discussion.

Next, based on the list of agreed qualities a relationship needs in order to thrive, create another diagram (see figure 12.3), this time together and including the qualities that *your particular relationship* needs. In this way, you get to apply the ideas you generated from a general discussion of relationships to something more specific to your particular situation and context. Anything that generates disagreement or discussion can be placed outside the relationship circle on the side of the partner who values it more.

Relationship Nourishment

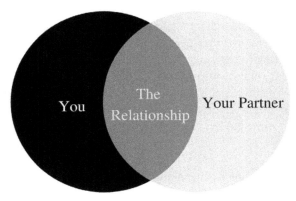

Figure 12.2.   Relationship nourishment.

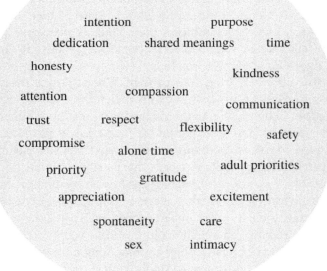

Figure 12.3.   Relationship qualities.

Once you have a collection of qualities you agree would nourish *your* relationship, you can then go about making some of those things priorities. It might be sending the kids off to grandma's house every other weekend so you can go bowling, have sex, or watch Netflix with a bottle of wine. Making time for that bondage class or dance class you've been meaning to attend, taking time to give and receive erotic massages, or practice caligraphy. It doesn't matter what it is, it just matters that you do it to nourish the relationship. When the sense of ease and compromise is practiced, it will be easier to practice negotiating sex and taking the sexual needs of the relationship into account too. This activity is designed to offer you a framework to think more objectively about your relationships and get a little refuge from the intensity that can come with renegotiating sexual habits.

Language, Lust, and Misunderstandings
Misunderstandings about sex, desire, our expectations of each other, and how sex is "supposed to" be often form the core of sexual problems in relationships. The problem is usually not sex but *communication* about sex and its offshoots—emotions, power, and turn-taking. Whether communication is verbal, physical, or even written is up to you, but without it, few erotic relationships can survive and be fulfilling. When left unattended for too long, bad sexual habits in relationships become the default. Poor sexual routines are at the center of most of our sex problems. But by now you know that the good news is that none of this is permanent and, with attention, it *can* be changed. The hump for a lot of us though is whether we really want change *that* much and / or how reasonable our expectations are. How dire do things have to get before something needs to be done? Are our expectations simply unrealistic and going to set ourselves up for disappointment? Engaging the Triangle of Satisfaction with curiosity, willingness, and priority, you'll discover what you need to know to make the changes you seek.

Case Study: Livinia and Keith
Livinia and Keith came to see me after two years of no sex. They met while traveling in South America and had been together for six years. When they met, Keith was high on the rush that travels brings, which can be as arousing and intriguing as the first flush of romance itself. For

Keith and Livinia, moving to suburban Melbourne after a year traveling together was like a benzo straight into Eros's heart. Keith fell back into business-as-usual being a Melbourne native, and Livinia took a blow to the soul, moving from her native Argentina all the way to Australia. So much was different for her, including the sex she was accustomed to having. She lamented that coming from Argentina where the pursuit of sex and seduction are cultural pastimes, she was unaccustomed to men not being as forward as they are in Argentina.

After the dust began to settle on their nuptials, Keith began chatting to women online, paying less attention to Livinia, then she slowly withdrew from him sexually. "I found out about the women online and I was hurt—but after a while I got over it. Now I believe him when he says he's not doing it anymore, but still, we're stuck."

"What do you think the problem is?" I asked.

There was silence.

Keith shifted in his seat, "Honestly, it was easier with the women online. They were keen and playful. It didn't matter, but with Liv, it matters. I give a shit what she thinks, so there's pressure."

"Pressure for what?" I was curious.

"To be good," he said. "To pleasure her. It's hard . . . I just . . . everything I do, she doesn't like."

Livinia interjected, "I tried to tell him what I liked, how to do it, how to touch me, but . . . he would just get upset. So we just stopped having sex altogether."

"And that was two years ago?" I confirmed.

"Yes. Two years," they agreed, glancing at each other.

"That's a long time to go without something you both want," I reflected. "So what's different now? Why do you want things to change?"

This is always a pivotal question in sex therapy. Like the "Why do you have sex?" question, "Why do you want things to change?" insists that you consider what you have, what you have lost and how far you are willing to go to get it back. It brings the power of sexuality back to you and invites you to reflect on the Triangle of Satisfaction with curiosity, willingness, and priorities.

"It's destroying our relationship," Keith said. "And it's my fault. I just don't know what to do in bed."

Liv continued, "It didn't make sense to me at the time, but I didn't realize how uncomfortable he was with sex, how insecure he was. Men in Argentina . . . ," she wavered a little, "I don't know, maybe they feel like that too, but with Keith, I was shocked. It took me months to understand that he was *really* telling the truth. I thought he was so handsome and confident . . . I mean how could he be so lacking in sexual confidence? It just doesn't make sense."

Between the two of them it was agreed that Keith's online shenanigans were inappropriate but, more than anything, it revealed that they had a big problem. And it wasn't just *having* sex; it was *communicating* about sex!

It turned out that Keith had no idea how to pleasure Livinia. And, worse still, he didn't know how to rectify that. And while she knew what she liked, she didn't know how to tell him. She had tried in the past, but Keith found it hard to hear. He took it as criticism and withdrew from her. She stopped trying and withdrew from him. It was around this time he started retreating to the safety of the women online. They required nothing from him and he had nothing to offer them. It was a perfect distraction. He felt accepted and secure in the anonymity of online interactions, which, while fun, eventually left him feeling empty. He longed to be sexually connected to Livinia but simply didn't have the knowledge or sexual and emotional intelligence to realize that her telling him how to touch her was a gesture of connection, not a criticism.

Both of them were trapped by the gendered expectations that men simply know (or are supposed to know) what they're doing sexually and women are not supposed to be assertive and ask for what they want. Confined by a lack of erotic knowledge and inefficient sexual communication, they were stranded—isolated from each other and feeling very much at the end of their ropes.

Although she loved Keith dearly, Livinia wondered how he'd managed sexually before meeting her, as he seemed timid, inexperienced, and frightfully unsure of himself in bed. In the beginning of their relationship, it was OK. They were both so keen to be in each other's company that the rush of finding time together offset the clumsy manoeuvres and awkwardness they felt discussing sexual preferences. But time and complacency created a recipe for intimidation and distress. For Livinia, Keith's reluctance to take the lead sexually was a stark contrast to how he was day-to-day. She'd started to wonder if he even still loved her. For her, love and sex were linked, whereas for Keith sex was a way of discovering love. Without an erotic atlas, he found himself shipwrecked. In previous relationships, sex mattered less; he was less invested emotionally, there was nothing to lose. There was no incentive to learn more than he knew, because he, like most people, simply thought sex was just about "sticking it in."

Keith's case is not rare. This lack of erotic wisdom underpins much of the suffering a vast majority of lovers experience sexually. Week in and week out I see the impact this has on couples who have been together anywhere from four months to forty years. When sex is reduced to erections, penetrations, and orgasms, it minimizes our capacity for pleasure, connection, and satisfaction. When we cannot express freely what we like and how we like to be touched, we are fated to a sex life that is as tedious and unfulfilling as it is painful.

In the case of Keith and Livinia, it almost cost their marriage. For both of them, having me provide the building blocks of (1) how to touch and (2) how her body worked to get more from sex took the sting out of not knowing. It reduced the shame of asking, listening, and having awkward conversations with each other. Instead, they had them with me. But for Keith, once that cat was out of the bag, it was a relief for him to get the tuition he needed to be able to move forward with greater confidence to please her.

Tolerating Unpleasant Touch

Many of us tolerate touch we don't want or enjoy. In many cultures though, it's a taboo to speak to it for fear of upsetting the "doer of the action" (Wheel of Consent in chapter 9). For Livinia, not enjoying the way Keith touched her didn't mean she didn't love him anymore. If anything, it meant she loved him enough to tell him the truth of how she was feeling and what she wanted.

From when we are young, we are told that to refuse touch is rude, inconsiderate, and may hurt someone's feelings. We are never taught how to assert what we like or how to respond when someone tells us what we are doing is not quite right for them. It can be tricky sometimes because a particular touch can feel good when we feel like it, while the

Time for Reflection

How do you feel about speaking up during sex? Asking for what you want? Saying what you don't want? Allowing? Enduring? Giving? Taking? Using the information that you gathered during the "Mindful Self-Pleasure Practice" in chapter 9 about what your body likes, what information might you be prepared to share with your partner or a potential partner about how you (generally) like to be touched? Look at your information from that practice and record yourself practicing what you might say and how you might say it.

next time it doesn't. If we don't speak up about what feels good and what doesn't, we are enduring touch rather than enjoying it, and nothing will change. But powerful forces stop like shame, stigma, a lack of education and skill prevent us from communicating what we like.

A build-up of resentment can lead to withdrawal, which was the case for Keith and Livinia. When anger and disappointment go unexpressed for too long, they can lead to the formation of bad habits and dissociation during sex. When we start tuning out from our bodies and our emotions, including the unpleasant ones like anger and resentment, we set ourselves up for tuning out from *all* of our sensations and emotions, including the pleasant ones like connection and desire. It's hard to get in the mood when you're busy tuning out of yourself and your feelings. And, as we learned in chapter 8, shame has a powerful impact on our ability to communicate about sex freely. When we resist expressing ourselves sexually because we judge our desires as weird or we fear being judged, being defective, not meeting expectations, or hurting another with our request, we limit the possibility for sexual transformation. If this resonates with you, go back to practicing the Three-Minute Game from chapter 9, taking turns following the course of both the action and the gift.

Low Libido versus High Libido
Couples usually have mismatched libidos at some stage in their relationship. This is not a red flag, nor is it the beginning of the end.

Despite its prevalence, this is an issue that couples find hard to navigate alone. The assumption is often that the partner with the lower libido is the one with the problem—that is, they are "frigid"—while the higher libido partner is not. When the higher libido is too high, that person is sometimes labeled a "sex addict" or "porn addict." Such useless and judgmental names from any point on the sexual spectrum offer nothing helpful. They merely reinforce stigma and shame around sexuality.

When clients come to me with a self-diagnosed low libido / high libido problem, I always ask what scale they used to diagnose their libido. The reality is that there is no medical or scientific scale for low libido or sex addiction. Broadly speaking, it's often women of all orientations that tend to diagnose themselves with low libido and often men of all orientations who get labeled by their partners as "sex addicts." It tends to have more to do with an objective moral compass than anything remotely connected to feeling good. These labels imply that there is some kind of sexual behavior going on that is problematic, either to the individual themselves, or within the relationship. But there is no scale for "normal" desire. It's simply a case-by-case situation that is a combination of sexual, personal, and relationship values, sexual practices, communication, and sexual integrity. In essence, "normal" is something we effectively make up as we go along. One person's normal is another person's shame; neither need be a tragedy.

In chapter 4, we considered the value of the frequency of sex. A lot of couples ask:

How often should we be having sex?
How often is normal?
What's the normal range?

The media comes up with a number. It's usually a decimal: 2.3 times a week or 1.7 times a week. We don't even know where this is coming from. Studies of sex are going to be determined by who we ask. Millennials in New York City will yield vastly different results from hill tribe people in Papua New Guinea. But which group offers a more accurate representation of human sexuality? Our sexual practices and values are profoundly affected by age, gender, religion, culture, ability, economics, access to technology, education, and many other variables.

Beyond this, it's hard to even determine what sex even is. Bill Clinton famously postulated this notion during his impeachment trial. Is oral sex, sex? Is cybersex, sex? Is anal sex, sex? What about BDSM? Or kissing? In order to determine concepts like "frequency" and "normal," we must ask ourselves what we are even talking about!

None of this is meant to suggest that libido differences are not a problem. They can be. Our libidos are not hardwired but may display variables that tend to be consistent. Some of us swing toward and away from sex at different times in our lives. I meet clients of all genders and orientations who describe a variety of attributes on the scale of low to high that affect their libido at different stages in their lives. These changes and fluctuations, while normal, can lead to problems when not managed and understood with compassion and knowledge. When there is a libido mismatch, there most definitely is a quest to be tended. Understanding that this is a shared quest is part of moving forward together. Good sex is not the responsibility of only one partner, it's created by both people, with understanding, generosity, and kindness.

But. . . . What Do I Say? How to Go About Telling and Listening
As much as it's great to understand the theory behind why we feel and do what we do in sex, it's normal to feel stumped by it too. The response from clients is often:

> Yeah, yeah, that's great. But, what can I say? Give me a script. How can I talk about this stuff with my partner?

or

> My partner is telling me all this, but what do I say back? I don't know how to respond to it.

Let's get practical again. There are times to speak and ways to speak, and the times and ways matter. Having more complex conversations about feelings and nuance are best done over lunch, dinner, in a car, or at the park rather than in bed in the middle of sex that's gone awry. This section will be about speaking about sex within your relationship, and the next about talking about sex in the middle of it—giving direction, if you will.

Talking about Sex When You're Not Doing It

Look back over all the notes and information you have gathered about yourself during the course of this book. All the "Time for Reflection" activities, all the questions you answered, all the "a-ha" moments you wrote in your notebook. All this data is your erotic template as it stands before you—*today*. It may change in a month or a year, but for today, this is it. You might like to present these research findings in a bar chart, a pie chart, a plot chart, a series of illustrations, photos, comic book strips, an essay, a short film, contemporary dance, a series of costumes—it's up to you. The main thing is that you start to take heed of this knowledge and practice using it and sharing it. Sharing what you have discovered about yourself and offering it up as a gift to help your relationship. If it feels overwhelming, go back chapter by chapter and take it a step at a time. It's a lot all at once. It might be easier to share about one chapter's worth of reflections at a time. There is no need to hurry any of this. What matters is that you speak about and share your ideas and desires. This is the "willingness" point on the Triangle of Satisfaction by taking the data from a page to an embodied practice.

Then when you have a sense of what you want to say and how you're going to say it, schedule a time to talk with your partner about it. Making sure you both have the time set aside is activating the "priority" point on the Triangle of Satisfaction. Nothing says "our sex life matters" more than scheduling time to talk about it.

When the time has come, decide who is going to speak first and who's going to listen first. If you aren't partnered, practice saying the following out loud or record yourself saying it.

Allow ten or fifteen minutes to describe what you would like to share for this session. If fifteen minutes is too long, try five minutes, or even two minutes. If you can talk for half an hour, that's okay too. Get a feel for what works for you. You don't need to stick rigidly to my suggestions. It's most important that you practice trusting yourself and your own limits and boundaries, without getting trapped by the brakes system (chapter 5) or the electric fence (chapter 10). If you do get trapped, recognize that it's happening. You can adopt the "curiosity" point on the Triangle of Satisfaction, by acknowledging the discomfort and asking yourself: *what might make it better right now?* Perhaps you need a break, so agree to put it aside for a moment and return after ten minutes or so. Remember, talking about sex in this way is best done at a time when you are not in the middle of sex or in the places where sex happens. Practicing talking about sex can happen just like talking about cooking, music, or films—just like things you like.

Some examples of how to start might be:

"I've been thinking about the kind of sex that I enjoy most with you and I really like . . . "
"I especially like it when we . . . "
"And I adore . . . "
"I like doing . . . "
"And I like receiving . . . "
"To me sex is important because . . . "
"And the reason I have sex or want to have sex is . . . "
"Sex for me is [name a few acts that you like] and I generally prefer [speed, timing, pressure]."

If this process feels difficult or clunky, that's OK. It is. Learning to communicate about sex feels difficult because we haven't been taught how to do it, it's not rewarded and there are no role models for it in our culture. It can make us feel vulnerable to communicate like this: both speaking and listening. No matter how advanced you are, keep it simple and keep it about yourself—and, as much as possible, start your statements about yourself and what you want with "I." Avoid starting sentences about sex with "you."

"I like it when you linger on my clitoris / balls / nipples / ass"

is much easier to hear than

"You always race to stick your fingers/dick into my pussy / ass. I hate that."

Or,

"You never spend enough time touching my clitoris / balls / nipples / ass."

It also provides a more useful framework than simply listing what you don't like. It's important to be clear about what you *don't* like, but that won't help your partner know what you *do* like.

Being a Better Listener

When it's your turn to listen, do so as if you are listening to an old friend. Or someone you have just met. Sometimes it's easier to have empathy for people who have lesser impact on us, or who aren't talking about *us* in their feelings. Imagine listening to your partner with curiosity (the Triangle again), rather than agenda. Practicing empathic listening is a really useful skill to develop when communicating sexual needs and longings. The idea is to listen with as little schema as possible. This can be very difficult when we're listening to somebody we have a vested interest in. Their thoughts, opinions, and our potential incompatibilities can be hard to hear when we want them to say things they may not be saying. Sometimes we can get caught up in what *we* want them to say, or how *we* want to respond to them, rather than *really* listening to them.

When discussing sex, a helpful habit to get into is saying "thank you" to acknowledge you have heard something they disclose, especially if there may be an element of sensitivity or vulnerability to it.

Responding with Helpful Questions

During or after the fifteen-minute speaking round, ask questions to get more understanding but do not judge, shame, or criticize. The intention is to get a better sense of what is actually important to your partner / self. For example, a statement might be:

> "I really like it when you whisper dirty stuff in my ear while you are playing with my clit."

And the response might be:

> "Ooooh, I am so glad to hear that, thanks for saying so. Is there anything in particular that I said that you really liked?"

If you aren't partnered, see if you have a friend who you would be willing to discuss sex with you (maybe more generally than the example above—or not).

Other responses could be:

"Tell me more about . . . "
"How was that for you?"
"What do/did you like about X?"
"How did it feel when X happened?"
"Would you like to change any part of that?"
"Would you like to do it again?"

When you are ready, change roles with the speaker becoming the listener and repeat. Use this framework as a guide any time you want to discuss sex, outside of sex time. The more you practice, the easier it becomes.

Speaking about Sex during Sex

I cannot emphasize enough how important it is to do the *heavy-lifting talking* about sex when you're not in the middle of it. There is nothing more challenging than trying to have a tender and vulnerable conversation with someone you care about when you're both nude, trying to impress, and, perhaps, with a bit of you inside a bit of them. Be kind to yourself and save the chatter during sex to be only about what's happening and what's feeling good, including requests to change or stop. But save the existential inquiry for other times, unless it's your "thing"—then, by all means, go for it.

When being given direction during sex, asking for confirmation / clarification is helpful, but keep the focus on consent and pleasure, without getting too wordy (unless you like that). A dialogue might sound like this:

"That's the spot, right there, now slow right down."
"Like this?"
"Slower still. . . . That's perfect. Stay right there. Yes! That's so good!"
"Thank you."

Such dialogue allows you to check speed or pressure when your partner / lover gives you some information about what they like. It is not only a way of letting them know it's OK to speak, but it also lets them know you have heard them and you acknowledge it. It generates easier communication than silence or endless apologizing.

The Sex Sandwich

One of the other strategies that is really helpful for talking about what you want—and can be used during sex—is something that I'm calling the Sex Sandwich (based on the idea of the Compliment Sandwich). The Sex Sandwich can be used during sex to aid erotic build up and play while still maintaining consent and communication and, more generally, to give feedback and make requests about things you might like to try or do differently

The slices of bread are two pieces of feedback that you like or are affirmative about your lover or a situation you are in. The sandwich filling is what you want. Mix and match and practice with these—not just in your head but out loud. Whether you are partnered or single, it can be extremely useful to get used to talking about sex out loud, stopping to notice how you feel when different words come out of your mouth. See these examples in table 12.1.

Affirmation (bread)	What You Want (filling)	Affirmation (bread)
• Oh my goodness, YES! • That feels so good! • You are so good at that! • I love it exactly like this! • This makes me so hard / wet / turned on! • I love hearing the sounds you make during sex!	• Pull my hair a little harder! • Got a condom? Are you ready? • Take me in your mouth—I love that! • Give it to me harder / softer / a little higher up! • Keep going just like that! • I really want to XXX right now. • Hearing this makes me want to XXX.	• That's it—so great. • I love fucking you! • Yes, just like that. • Mmmm—this is perfect. Thank you! • I love how you look / sound / feel when we XXX. • Hearing you and XXXing drives me crazy.

The Sex Sandwich can be used during regular sex conversations, away from bed, to discuss general ideas and requests or, more specifically, if you are doing something you both agreed to and you want to change it up a little. During sex, when something feels good, give that feedback:

"Oh, I love that."
"That's the spot."
"I love it when you . . . "
"That really turns me on."

These kinds of things are particularly helpful as the closing bread on the sandwich.

If receiving direction is a challenge for you, invite curiosity (Triangle) and try "allowing" it (Wheel of Consent) as a gift and not as a criticism. Recognize that they're telling you what they want, not because you are inadequate but because they want to create a better sexual connection with you and they want things to change. Without that free flow of information, it's just not going to happen.

If you are asked for something that is really uncomfortable for you, stop there and ask:

"Ooooh, that sounds great, but not right now. Is there something else that you would like?"

Remember, just because it's asked for, doesn't mean it has to be given. Kindness and generosity are the key here. If you start feeling so uncomfortable that you are no longer present, you're tuning out or simply enduring it, STOP! Recalibrate and try again another time. You have permission to stop sex whenever necessary. Discussions can happen later.

Addressing Difficulties after Sex

Sex is awkward. Maybe not every time, but often enough. This doesn't mean that you are doomed, nor does it mean there is something fundamentally wrong. Many times, therapeutic discussions with clients center on dismantling and accommodating the awkwardness of sex. Getting used to being a little uncomfortable, especially when trying new things, is completely normal and nothing to worry about, but these things *do* need to be addressed from time to time.

Sometimes when a partner is reluctant to discuss sex, it's not always sex that is the issue but, rather, their fears or concerns that you are unhappy with them as a person. Many people take sexual preferences and requests personally, when, in other situations, they would not. If a partner tells you they don't like blueberry pie, it's not because *you* made it—they simply don't like the sweet fruit and would not enjoy it no matter who makes it. Yet with sex, conversations can get derailed when expressing the same limitations because talking about sex is very personal. A lot of people find it very difficult to distinguish *how* they are sexually with *who* they are as a person.

If you say, for example, "I like being bitten a little, especially on the neck," the listener might not hear that. They may be too caught up in their own situation and not fully listening to the statement being made as a piece of information. Instead they may hear, "I like biting—(which means I don't like you.)" Their internal monologue may respond with, *I'm not into biting so I'm just going to remove myself from this conversation.* They respond as if it were a criticism rather than an invitation for conversation. If this is the situation, it can be helpful to remind them that you are not criticizing but offering information about yourself as a means of deepening connection. They may also simply feel too inexperienced to manage such conversations, in which case, a gentle approach is necessary, possibly with the help of a skilled therapist or coach.

Another reason people struggle to talk about sex is that they feel they have tried and they haven't been heard. In the situation with Livinia and Keith, Keith struggled to hear what Livinia was saying without getting caught up in his own lack of confidence. None of these things are insurmountable, but they do take practice. Remember to practice being a better listener by asking questions that expand the conversation, not shut it down. This encourages more discussion and allows the speaker to feel heard.

If what's being asked of you during sex is not possible, invite a request for something else or offer something else, then talk about it later, when you're not having sex. Save it for the next day.

Reschedule

The Triangle of Satisfaction requires prioritizing. If your partner says, "Can we talk about sex? This is important to me," or there was an awkward moment the day before during sex, discuss it. It's important that you have the time and the energy for such conversations, so agreeing to a time is important. When things unexpectedly crop up, acknowledge them and offer an alternative time. Don't be afraid to say, "Now is not a good time," if it's really not a good time. If you're distracted, tired, hungry, or about to go out the door, say, "I want to talk about this. But now is not a good time. Let's talk about it tomorrow." If you say, "Let's talk about it tomorrow," then honor that. Acknowledge that the conversation is important and if you need to reschedule, take it upon yourself to do that rather than burden the other with that responsibility. Avoid scheduling a time and then just abandoning it, thinking, "If I forget about it then it won't happen." That's not fair. Connection is built on trust.

But I'm Still Stuck . . .

If you are looking for ways to connect more deeply and to bring more passion to your relationships, it's important that you try to create a container to hold space for such intimacy. Yet sometimes, no matter how much you build safe containers and try to have conversations and you're really doing the best that you can to listen and speak, they still just don't go anywhere. Some days you're still met with or experience some kind of resistance, shame, brakes, or electric fences. Try leaving it for a few days, possibly for a few weeks. Bashing away can sometimes make it worse. Remember Mel and Chris from chapter 10: too much processing can weigh heavily on eroticism.

And then again, if there's still no response, or there's still no effort coming in from the other side in relation to these questions and practices, it could possibly be time for you to reconsider how important sex is to you in this particular relationship.

- What might it be like to allow yourself to not be sexual for a while?
- What might it be like to allow this relationship to not be sexual at all?

- What does the relationship bring you in other ways?
- If this situation were not to change, would that be OK with you?

Flexibility is key here, as is a gentle degree of self-inquiry. You may also really benefit from finding a therapist to help you.

In the next and final chapter, we'll take a pragmatic look at some of the most common issues people face when navigating desire issues in their relationships and what to do about them as we tie all the pieces together.

CHAPTER 13

Troubleshooting

Like failure, chaos contains information that can lead to
knowledge—even wisdom.

—Toni Morrison

In this final chapter, we'll practice orienting ourselves toward pleasure
and integrity in a culture that benefits from us remaining untethered
from our source. There are many reasons why lovers find themselves
stuck when it comes to sex and intimacy. Whether a lack of knowledge,
a lack of priority, a lack of consideration, a lack of resources, a lack of
practice, sensitivity, ignorance, stubbornness, shame, complex personal
histories, a lack of interest, or simply differences in desires or libido, it's
well established that maintaining sexual enthusiasm both in and out of
relationships can be challenging. This is due, in part, to two foundational elements of human sexuality: meaning and eroticism. But before
we get into that, let's consider some of the most common reasons we
may need to troubleshoot our libido.

Reasonable Reasons People Who Used to Like Sex Stop Wanting It
Throughout this book I haven't really spent any time looking at some of the biomedical reasons people may begin to lose interest in sex. While these reasons are relevant, I have deliberately excluded them for two reasons: one, is it's not my wheelhouse and I'm unqualified to offer medical advice; and two, the medical approach to sex tends to focus very heavily on performance over pleasure and by now you know pleasure is something we can all access how, when, and if we want to.

That said, the list below, while not exhaustive, offers common reasons people may temporarily disconnect from their libido and overall enthusiasm for pleasure. Understandably, many of these issues will affect not only sex, but general quality of life.

- hormone imbalances
- grief
- guilt and shame
- fear of expressing unacceptable emotions
- distrust or fear of partner
- discovery of partner's infidelity
- boredom
- suppressing unfulfilled desires
- abuse or past history of abuse
- autoimmune problems
- metabolic imbalances
- hormonal contraceptives
- lack of sex education
- lack of communication
- lover who doesn't or won't offer pleasure
- no longer attracted to partner
- not having a sexual partner
- not having regular arousal and orgasm (partnered or solo)
- societal message that you shouldn't be enjoying sex due to age, gender, orientation, preference, religion, etc.
- job stress or job loss
- financial problems
- relationship stress
- conflict with partner
- relationship staleness
- lack of sexual variety
- illness
- side effect of medication
- depression
- anger
- lack of exercise
- poor eating choices
- overuse of alcohol or recreational drugs
- low self esteem
- low self-image

Some of these have been addressed throughout this book while others, more rooted in pathology and medical issues, have not; yet, they still benefit from applying the tools and the wisdom gleaned within your erotic template. When overall health and medical issues seemingly unrelated to sex affect us, they can and do have an effect on quality of life and sometimes desire. But like Ed in chapter 12, illness, biological changes, and aging are not immediately the death knell to one's sex life. These reasons will apply to those in very specific contexts at very specific times. When struggling with medical issues, understand that the effect on your sex life will make itself known, but how you manage it depends upon many things including your personal values and conditions and the communities you inhabit that remind you that your pleasure matters.

When Sex Just Doesn't Come Easy

When partners experience disruptions in their sex lives, there are always a wide range of reasons, many of which include responses to our erotic template's conditions and contexts not being realized or embodied. Such conditions and contexts may be emotional, physical, psychological, cultural, or derived from some internal process that needs further unpacking to determine the best way through. While there is never one true path, many long for a one-size-fits-all method, a sure-fire way to avoid complexity and arrive at the most mind-blowing sex ever by just pressing a button. Sadly, eroticism doesn't work like that. Eroticism exists where our creativity takes flight. Imagination and possibility propel us toward new adventures, but our minds and bodies may have other ideas. Surrender is an essential ingredient, but is the nemesis of control. Surrendering to *what is* doesn't mean giving up but, instead, working *with* what's happening rather than against it. Take Lewis from chapter 8, for example. As an officer of the law, his body was having a very reasonable response to threat and danger. The trouble was, the response had become a habitual default rather than a choice. In this instance, Lewis' willingness (Triangle of Satisfaction) to surrender to the truth of the situation and begin to learn to change his relationship to his body, allowed him to move closer to the sex life he desired. Had he fought, resisted, and cock-blocked himself with a refusal to soften or work with the issue somatically, he may not have found the resolutions he was after. This was a grand effort of both him and his partner, and his capacity to engage the totality of his being— body, mind, and heart.

This is true of those who steadfastly hold the idea that sex should be spontaneous or that they must feel horny for sex to proceed. When we rely on the body alone to propel us forward, we may find ourselves stuck, frozen, or numb, just like Maze way back in chapter 4. When horniness doesn't descend as we've been taught, we think there's something wrong with *us* rather than the model we've consumed. The complexity of *wanting to want* is hard, no doubt. The mind wants to lose control but the body won't allow it, or vice versa. Without exploration, the tension between the imagination, the body, and the heart can turn sex into a warzone; one we'd rather abandon for the calmer waters of domesticity and familiarity.

Tension is a paradox. It's at once a source of anxiety and also the rebirth we seek. Much of what eroticism requires is our ability to tolerate and explore tension and uncertainty. In many ways, it's about finding the balance between tension and intimacy. Too far one way or the other, and we lose our grip on the precious gift we revere. The difficulty is in tolerating the discomfort long enough to allow the knowledge to appear. It's easy for us to balk at the usual advice about the importance of communication. Even if we *know* it is the foundation of so much of what's important in creating great relationships and sexual connections. But so many of us do not do it. We know better, but we just do not act. The problem is that there are a variety of reasons that speaking up about sex doesn't happen, and without discussing them, we are in danger of bypassing the painful feelings and experiences that help us make changes.

Many of the reasons we resist change are about self-preservation. We want to avoid shame and embarrassment or are concerned a fight will start. There's fear that we are abnormal or weird. A lot of us do not know what we like or how to ask for it, or believe that this is "just how sex is." But in order to create change, we have to believe, first and foremost, there is another way, a better way. Without this, it's hard to find the courage to make changes and move forward. We have to believe that the effort is worthwhile, and we have to work as a team for the relationship to shift course.

Case Study: Gavin and Tracey

Gavin and Tracey had been together for eighteen years when they came to see me during a period of very intense trouble in their relationship. They loved each other but the relationship was well and truly under a lot of strain.

Tracey worked full time as a teacher and Gavin had his own business in construction. They both enjoyed their work but agreed that their sexual relationship had been neglected for far too long. Things had started going poorly for them when they realized conceiving a baby through intercourse was not going to be possible. Tracey had had several rounds of IVF, which took a toll on her physically and on both of them emotionally. Despite their best efforts, conception simply never happened and, instead, they chose to adopt.

The troubles in their sex life started becoming a real problem with the pressure of conception. In many ways, the issues were actually right there from the start but were simply considered "normal" and nothing to worry about.

Over the years, sex became "robotic," in their words. It started with trying to conceive. They were having sex by the calendar and this routine stuck. Neither of them looked forward to sex because it had—quite frankly—"become insufferable." All creativity and enthusiasm had gone and sex was very much about getting pregnant rather than getting close or getting off. And they were angry. Really angry. They were supposed to be in love. They were supposed to loving the idea of getting pregnant. Why were things simply not working?

They were so overwhelmed by the desire to conceive that these emotions became focused on each other rather than the problem itself.

It's hard to understand a tapestry of complex emotions when you are experiencing lots of conflicting emotions at the same time.

- How is it possible to love someone and resent them?
- How is it possible to want sex with someone you are angry with?
- How is it possible to bring this up when you are unsure of the meaning of your own feelings?

For a lot of couples, when sex issues come up it can be extremely hard to navigate them. Many of us don't know how to talk about sex, let alone the strain of external circumstances like starting a family. Many people lack the skills to talk about *anything* complex and emotional effectively, and this is often when problems sit and fester for years. This is exactly what had happened to Gavin and Tracey.

Misunderstanding + Poor Sex Education = Disaster
Gavin was thoroughly confused by Tracey's apparent lack of desire for him. More than anything he wanted her to *want* him, and she did . . . but in ways that he wasn't recognizing. Like most people, Gavin believed that desire had to come before arousal (chapter 4), and that Tracey had to be turned-on to pursue him. Sex had gone from something fun when they were dating, to pressure and a race against the clock when they were trying to conceive. That, combined with hormonal upheavals and sex's association with conception, made discussing sex taboo—a source of shame and sadness for both of them. Instead of exploring these darker emotions, they were misplaced upon each other and humbly pushed down and ignored.

Years after the children finally came into their lives, sex was still taboo but for different reasons. It was no longer a source of sadness but, rather, a void that called to be filled with neither of them knowing how.

Tracey had always believed that sex had to be about feeling horny, and because she wasn't, she was able to push it aside. Gavin simply didn't know that Tracey's desire for him could be stimulated in ways that were not just physical. Although she had tried to tell him, he didn't hear her because the idea was so foreign to him. This, combined with the complexity he felt between longing for Tracey and being mad at her, made it difficult for him to really comprehend her sexual needs. He was so caught up in trying to look for familiar clues of desire that he didn't see or hear the signals she was trying to offer him.

Beyond this, Tracey lacked the confidence to discuss sex explicitly, which bewildered Gavin. In many ways she was the confident one in the relationship—the driver, the organizer, the boss—but, when it came to sex, she would clam up and simply couldn't say what she wanted. She knew what she liked, sort of, but the expanse between telling him what she wanted and feeling like he didn't "get it" was simply too great to bear.

Gavin was tuned in to only spontaneous desire and she was displaying all the signs of responsive desire (chapter 5) but lacked the skills to tell him. This continued for years before they came to see me. They gave up on each other; but, neither told the other.

They did it with their actions.

They stopped connecting.

It wasn't until several sessions in that they noticed their antagonism toward each other sounded like they had both abandoned the relationship and each other—but neither was talking about it.

Gavin told me in detail how much of a control freak Tracey was. She managed everything, she was so sure of everything, and he admired her and resented her for it too. If she was so together, why couldn't she control her sexuality also? Why couldn't she just make herself want him the way he wanted her? He was tired of asking and tired of waiting. For someone who had her act together like she did, he couldn't help but take it personally. He was offended. He was hurt. He was lonely. He was missing her. He was also utterly at a loss as to how to be different for her.

Tracey was furious with him. She thought he was a lazy and selfish lover, obsessed only with himself and having orgasms. In the session, she broke down sobbing. Gavin was mortified. In his mind, he had been accommodating to her needs. Why was she so upset? Why was she doing this to him?

She wasn't doing anything *to him*. It's what she *wasn't* doing that was contributing to the problem. She was so shy talking about sex that she simply never told him she needed him to *slow down*. His rushed approach to sex was what turned her off. All this time she thought she was abnormal for not liking intercourse much. This sense of feeling abnormal, coupled with the wish that he would just slow the whole thing down and give her time to get turned on, sat at the heart of her resistance toward him, but also toward sex. She realized she had been blaming him for not being a good lover when, in fact, she also thought *she* was abnormal and a lousy lover. Her lack of sexual knowledge preceded her and clouded her ability to see things for what they really were.

Gavin was stunned. He thought he had been doing "the right thing." His sex education, like most Western men of that generation, was rudimentary at best. The focus was on erections, intercourse, and his orgasm as a symbol of a successful liaison. He was being manly, powerful, and having sex like they always had. She liked that at the start, but something had changed. Tracey's upbringing meant she was uncomfortable discussing sex. Her sex education at school didn't cover pleasure, and, despite being vocal in other areas of life, she didn't know she had the right to ask. Her friends would brag about how great their sex lives were and Tracey retreated further into herself. She internalized the shame of not enjoying sex and had no idea how to make changes.

It was not until their relationship was on the brink of separation that they decided to come to see me. They had let it get *that bad* before intervening. Retrospectively, they both realized they could have changed things much earlier.

The Path Out of Darkness
Over time, Gavin learned to make sex more about Tracey. She anxiously showed him how she masturbated (which ended up being one of their favorite shared activities). He didn't realize she could orgasm without penetration, nor did he realize smaller, gentler movements were actually more powerful for her. He had been so caught up in being "manly" that it simply never occurred to him that his anxiety could have been rectified by simply slowing everything right down.

Gavin also conceded that he really could do more in terms of taking the load off Tracey by arranging the kids' events and allowing her more time for herself. She was able to relax more and let go of her "control freak" persona, which was activating her brakes and making her anxious and distressed about sex. Once she had time to slow down and focus on herself, sex ceased to be another chore on her to-do list and, instead, became an opportunity to relax a little.

Things started going well for Gavin and Tracey. Gavin arranged date nights every week, including taking care of babysitting arrangements. They were spending quality time together and made a point of practicing being nice to each other. They recognized that they had fallen into some really bad habits of striking out at each other with their anger. By paying more attention to the kind of relationship and sex they wanted, they were learning to think before they spoke and were mindful of the effect such actions had on the closeness they both so sorely craved. Gavin still struggled to really come to terms with Tracey's conditions for sex being linked to relaxation and time rather than lust, but he recognized that for them to be intimate, this was non-negotiable.

They were having sex around once a week and, when I quizzed them about it, they both reported that they were actually enjoying it. They finally understood that what made it better was communicating meaningfully about what they wanted.

Feeling the Feels

Two of the most common emotions that stop us talking about sex are shame and fear—primal, deep emotions. Core emotions that dwell within the lizard brain and, when activated, affect our brakes by putting them in overdrive when we feel overwhelmed or confused about sex and intimacy, just like Tracey.

Globally renowned shame researcher Brené Brown defines shame as:

> the intensely painful feeling or experience of believing that we are flawed and therefore unworthy of love and belonging—something we've experienced, done, or failed to do makes us unworthy of connection.[1]

Let's consider the impact of this in a sex context. When shame gets in the way, nothing else survives. The insidious nature of shame is so treacherous that it has the ability to destroy even the most loyal and loving connections. The trouble with shame in sex is that it can have the effect of altering our identity, like it did with Tracey (*I am a bad and broken person*), as well as reducing our capacity for pleasure and connection (*I cannot say what I like because I am a bad and broken person*). Instead of seeing ourselves as "good people" experiencing a shame response to a sexual context, it's easy to fuse with the shame and believe it is *part of us* rather than something we are experiencing in that moment. Remember the case of John (chapter 11) with the intrusive thoughts of his past partners and images he saw in porn while he was having sex with his current partner? He thought *he* was at fault. He, like Tracey, fused with the intrusive thoughts and thought that *he* was a "bad person" rather than a person *experiencing a shame response to* something that was quite normal and pleasurable. Almost every single case study in this book shares this core issue in common. They all believed that they were flawed based on the myths and beliefs they've inherited about sex and how it's supposed to be. They fused with the story of their flawed essence so much that they were convinced *they* were the problem. I believe the reason for this being such a widespread phenomenon is cultural. Culturally, speaking about sex out loud *is* a shameful act. Having sex, in a committed, monogamous relationship is OK, but speaking about it out loud, not so much. Traditionally, too much discussion of sex gets you labeled a "pervert"; another in the pile of rejects nobody wants near them, because shame is and has always been an extremely effective tool for social control. Perverts, sex addicts, the emasculated, sluts, and whores are among the refugees of a society unable to deal with the complexity of human sexuality. Without the freedom to speak out, our uncomfortable feelings are internalized. In other words, our uncomfortable feelings have nowhere to go but stay within us and they grow there and fester like a tumor. When this happens, we do not "own" them. Instead, we *become* them. When this happens, we keep ourselves small and silent to avoid disturbing them. If we can just keep them under control, we may fly under the radar and no one will know just how "bad" we are.

When people feel bad about *who* they are to their core, it's easier to manipulate and coerce them into silence or tolerating the intolerable. Sadly, sex falls into this category because there are just so few contexts in which explicit discussions about sex are encouraged. Even Brené Brown, the doyen whose brilliant work on shame is revolutionary, avoids discussing sex in depth and at length. Because there is little to no frame of reference for speaking about sex, its silence renders it a taboo. We get fooled into thinking it's not important, which drives shame further underground. When we feel afraid that we are the only ones feeling what we feel about sex, it's easy for fear to transform into shame, where it wreaks havoc slowly but surely on our sex lives and our relationships.

Shame in a sexual context, manifests in a variety of ways, from keeping us small and silent, through to more extreme versions of dissociation, checking out, feeling unworthy, disconnected and going numb. It alters our perception of ourselves and each other. When we are operating from under the cloud of shame, it can feel like there is no way out because we are convinced that we are the ones at fault. That's how shame keeps its hold on us. Likewise, fear can be debilitating, especially when we do not know what we are afraid of. Being afraid of ourselves, of our partners, of liking something you saw in porn, of trying something new (in case you like it), of being broken or of getting our comeuppance. Fear, like shame, is a strong activator of the electric fence. It keeps us way back from stepping over the edge. Worst of all, fear eliminates curiosity. It's hard to remain curious when you are afraid. It removes the stability from the Triangle of Satisfaction, transforming the most stable structure on Earth to something unreliable and untrustworthy.

We can always find an excuse not to change. Change can be scary. Sex can be scary. Part of embracing the change we seek is in learning to acknowledge, with all that we are, that what we have been told about sex is a lie. We must learn, instead, to replace this lie with the wisdom within us, our unique and personal way through. But first we must tune into it.

Suggestion: Reread chapters 2, 6, 7, and 8. Reflect on your responses to "Times for Reflection."

Checking-Out

Checking-out of sex and intimacy is often a direct result of shame and fear. It can also be the result of trauma, which has its own category below. Checking-out can take many forms. Some of the more common ones include going blank, holding your breath, not moving much or at all, thinking excessively about other things, using fantasy to endure touch you don't like or that hurts, getting distracted by anything else in the room or getting swept up with the chatter in your mind. There are many more but these are the most common.

More advanced ways of checking out are developing a heavy reliance on overanalyzing ourselves, also known as "staying in our heads," dependence upon fantasy and excessive porn consumption—where the focus is less on creating synergy between partners and more on building an escape to avoid sensation, vulnerability, or reality. To clarify, I am absolutely in favor of using porn and fantasy to enhance our sex lives. I also enjoy rigorous mental self-inquiry. But like anything good, when used recklessly, as a crutch, and without integrity it can be the catalyst for angst in our lives. Moderation and mindfulness are the key.

When we check out during sex, it stops us from being accountable. It's what happens when we let the "allowing" quadrant from the Wheel of Consent (chapter 9) dominate our sexual interactions rather than speaking up for what we want (chapter 12). It stops us from having to take notice of our feelings and sensations in the moment (chapter 8). It means we can avoid feeling anything at all and eliminates the obligation to communicate about it, like Tracey. This is why checking out can be a strong default for couples who find communicating about sex difficult, have got stuck in a rut or find themselves resentful. When checking out during sex becomes the go-to to get through sex, things need to change. When we avoid tending to our feelings during sex, we make it impossible for ourselves or our partners to create connection, because *we are not there*. When fantasy becomes a tool to avoid the present situation, it can actually increase your body's sense of enduring unwanted touch. Your body is still receiving something it doesn't want, while your mind is elsewhere. That reinforces the somatic programming that says that this is "something to be tolerated" rather than something to be changed.

Suggestion: Reread chapters 2, 8, 9, and 12. Practice staying with the sensations in your body while arousal builds. Sometimes it can be helpful to speak what you're feeling in a constant narrative—with a willing partner this can be a helpful way to practice staying focused. Also consider hiring professional bodyworkers to assist with staying present during complex sensations.

Technical Difficulties

Sometimes what contributes to a low desire and mismatched libidos is ineffective sexual technique. Such issues can actually be really easily addressed and are no one person's fault. Whether accomplished lovers or novices, we still need to pay attention to what we are doing and who the touch is for (chapter 9). Troubles set in when the sex we are having doesn't feel good to one or both of us anymore. Sometimes it's because we get stuck in our own nervous system, like Lewis (chapter 8). Many of us will get stuck here and find it hard to speak up about what we want (chapter 12). We can be afraid of upsetting our partner by asking them to do something different, especially if we have toler-ated something we didn't like for a long time just to keep the peace. After a time though, these feelings make us feel worse and an honest yet compassionate conversation can be really helpful in recalibrating what's going wrong. Remember, it's your responsibility to speak up if sex isn't working out for you as much as it's your responsibility to listen when your partner tells you they need sex to be done differently, like Gavin and Tracey. In the moment, use the Sex Sandwich (chapter 12) but, if shame holds you hostage, seek a therapist or coach for support.

Suggestion: Reread chapters 8, 9, and 12. Do the erotic massages. Use the scripts. Get used to the discomfort of talking about sex. Go to my website for other resources to help you learn more about touching, our bodies, and pleasure.

Resentment, Frustration, and Other Unresolved Emotional Conflict

Unresolved emotional conflict can be very destructive to our relation-ships and our sex lives. Over time, little things become big things and can shut down otherwise great partnerships. Learning to feel your emotions, distinguish thoughts from feelings, practicing listening and responding, knowing your triggers, and practicing how to communicate effectively are essential life skills that I urge everyone to undertake no matter what. Investing in such potent wisdom changes the trajectory of your emotional satisfaction in your relationships and your life.

Unchecked and unacknowledged emotions have a way of shutting down our capacity to enjoy pleasure. To cope, we might start tolerat-ing unwanted or unpleasant touch. Over time, our capacity for pleasure becomes virtually zero. Trying to rationalize our way through hurt feel-ings is never helpful, nor is having dramatic reactions to feelings that are fresh and activated. Without some degree of good feeling toward your partner, or at least faith that things are changing and looking up, it can be hard to cultivate any aspects of the Triangle of Satisfaction (chapter 7) when we are shut down and angry.

That resentment ripples out into the rest of your life. You have less resilience when difficult things happen. When miscommunications and conflicts arise, you're less able to assume that the other person has good intentions and you jump to conclusions about their motiva-tions. Carrying the internal pain of resentment might make you lash out at others or it might make you pull away. Such black and white thinking can often be a response to trauma, so it's important to address emotional complexities head on. However it plays out, the resentment that forms from remaining silent or enduring unwanted touch, affects everything else you experience and do.

When resentment and enduring sex become the norm, most people pick one of two choices: they avoid sex entirely or they dissociate. Dissociation, like checking out, is a protective strategy because it removes your awareness from the unpleasant situation you find yourself in, but, long-term, it's a disaster for your relationships and your sex life.

Suggestion: Consider taking courses in couples' communication or hiring a therapist, coach, or counselor who is highly experienced in couples work. Drop the BS and ask yourselves sincerely: Do you *want* to move past the frustrations or is there some payoff to remaining resentful? For example, Do you get to control your partner? Do you get revenge? What does staying frustrated and resentful make possible? What does staying frustrated and resentful shut down or minimize? If you were not frustrated and resentful, what could you be instead? Practice acting that out just to see how it feels. Get counseling if you need support. Resentment is poison. Do not let it fester.

Lack of Trust

In hookups, paid transactions, or casual encounters, trust is primarily established by engaging in clear conversations that center consent and willingness. This also applies in established romantic relationships; however, the significant difference is *how* your partner responds to your requests and offers takes on greater importance. The more you are in the relationship the more vulnerable you are. Having sex with people you don't know or much care about can be easy. When love merges with sex, it can become at once intoxicating and dangerous because suddenly trust and the potential for betrayal become relevant. Trust isn't just a concept we read about. It's a subjective experience that must be embodied and felt over and over again. When trust is experienced in this way, the relationship provides a secure container and opportunities for depth and connection including with sex. Mutual trust can then take a back seat, humming along in the background, allowing lovers the platform from which to take risks both emotionally and sexually.

But if this container is cracked, anxieties and insecurities awaken. The intensity of these feelings may intrude periodically, or cover the entire relationship. In order for intimacy to be reestablished, trust needs to be rebuilt so that quality sex can emerge.

Conditions That Build Trust
- accepting / encouraging
- sensitive / concerned
- emotionally open
- responsive / engaged
- committed / reliable

Conditions That Corrode Trust
- critical / judgmental
- aloof / indifferent
- defensive / closed-off
- unresponsive / detached
- erratic / unpredictable

The conditions take of a variety of meanings when they come from a person you care for. The loved partner wields the power and influence to help you feel secure and connected as well as insecure and anxious. When trust is broken, couples shift from secure to insecure / anxious modes of relating, including anger and withdrawal. Because sex in an intimate partnership is inherently more emotionally risky than other environments, it at once holds the potential to induce the richest tenderness and vulnerability, and, when conditions are not met, emotional wounding and withdrawal. And as previously established in chapter 9, good intentions are rarely enough to make things always work the way we need them to. Hoping that things just simply "work out," in my experience, is mere folly. For sex that's worth wanting, intention matters as much as emotional skill building and practice.

Include the trust conditions above in your conversations about erotic conditions and personal values (chapter 6) alongside erotic values (chapter 12) where relevant, especially when trust has been corroded. A lack of trust in relationships can make satisfying sex harder to access and the Triangle of Satisfaction obsolete. If the trust issue is due to a situation(s) that happened within this relationship, sometimes that needs to be addressed and repaired before sex can start to heal. If the trust issues are historical / trauma related, counseling and / or somatic trauma therapy is advised and strongly encouraged.

Suggestion: What is the source of the trust problem? Your partner? The situation? Yourself? Someone's history? It's amazing how many partners try to heal sexual rifts without first identifying the problem. From there, it's easier to address the elephant in the room. What might create trust for the wounded partner? What boundaries exist about this situation? How will they be honored between you? Be specific about what they are and how you will manage a violation of boundaries should it occur. Having a plan for emotional management in tense situations is helpful and much of this is best done under the facilitation of a skilled professional.

Aging, Poor Health, and Injury

Poor health, both mental and physical, can dampen one's enthusiasm for sex at times, while for others, like Ed (chapter 12), it can create a fervor not seen before. Depending upon the issues you are experiencing, there are a host of professionals able to support you in navigating sex and pleasure under complex circumstances. Sometimes you just need information; other times you need practice and skill. It can be challenging talking to medical professionals about pleasure because, while they are trained in medicine, they are often not trained in well-being and pleasure. Learning how to speak up with health providers is as essential as learning to speak up with partners and lovers. My friend and colleague Joan Price, advocate for ageless sexuality,[2] suggests we must get used to life in our new bodies when we experience changes due to injury, illness, and aging.

Suggestion: Seek support groups for sexuality that focus on your particular issue. Look for them online. There is a support group for virtually everything these days, including your condition and its intersections with sex and pleasure. Do not underestimate the value of a supportive community of restoring faith in your sex life. Beyond this consider: Can you help manage the situation by changing diet, medication, or exercise? Can you change your practices to suit your new situation? For example, prostatectomy often means softer erections but needn't mean no sex. Take workshops in erotic massage, oral sex, and mutual masturbation to discover how to pleasure penises in all stages of life. Same applies to vulvas post-partum or post-menopause. All bodies change as they age or as a result of accident or illness. Transformation is inevitable, so we must learn to adapt. Consider: What is possible for you sexually right now? Are you *willing* to experiment with what's possible? Apply the Triangle of Satisfaction (chapter 7) to the conditions and values (chapters 6 and 12) you have identified as possible.

Anxiety and Depression

Traditionally it was understood that both anxiety and depression were libido killers. And while for some this may be true, my friend and colleague Jo Ellen Notte, mental health advocate and author of *The Monster Under the Bed: Sex, Depression and the Conversations We Aren't Having*,[3] suggests that while these conditions are cause for pause, they alone are not the reason people's sex lives suffer. While researching her book, she discovered that couples affected by depression and anxiety who reported high sexual satisfaction were couples who learned to communicate about it meaningfully. In other words, these couples didn't let their conditions overwhelm them. Instead, they were proactive in finding ways to incorporate sex into their relationships on good days, and communicated about it regularly to make sure all parties' needs were being met as best as possible. While a perfect sex life is never the goal, finding solutions that work, outside of the box, is helpful.

Suggestion: Look back over your sexual conditions and values (chapters 6 and 12). Also take another look at the Triangle of Satisfaction (chapter 7). Lifting yourself up when you're feeling down can feel risky. Take another look at chapter 10. Are there times where you are more likely to feel like sex? If so, what kinds of sex? Are there times where you feel more confident communicating about sex? Are there situations in which sex feels less burdensome? Discuss these with your partner. Work within the specific limitations that sex brings for you within this context. If your anxiety is in response to a specific sexual context, try the Three-Minute Game as a framework to move it through with your partner. Practice asking for touch that you like, not that you tolerate. Get clear on *why* you're doing sex and what you're doing. Practice staying present and not checking out, as above.

Mindfulness has been proven to be an extremely effective treatment for anxiety-related sex problems, though for some it can make the symptoms worse. If so, I recommend working with a somatic practitioner, either in person or virtually, to learn new ways of being with the body during episodes of anxiety in connection with arousal.

Avoiding Disappointment / Being Disappointing

Emotions in relationships can be hard. Sad but true. As we learned in chapter 3, love and desire are often really different, and the messages we receive about love and romance are nearly as damaging as the messages we receive about sex. Learning to manage emotions is a key skill in creating and sustaining magnificent relationships, both sexual and platonic. Longing to be on the same page as your partner is common. In an ideal world, our emotions—including our libidos and desires—would be in sync all the time. But they are not. And this is normal. Longing for your desire or your partner's desire, over time, can become anti-desire if left unchecked. And if historically you have avoided talking about or engaging in sex to avoid your or your partner's disappointment, it can be hard to shift that.

Consider the difference between,

"You disappointed me when you told me you didn't enjoy oral sex,"

and,

"I feel disappointment when I realize that our sexual palettes are different."

These two phrases, while not identical, both deal the core emotion of disappointment. However, while the first frames the subject (you) as the source of the problem (e.g., "you do this to me"), the second allows the subject "I" to be the center, and the experience of "disappointment" is a subjective response to a disappointing context—*our palettes are different*. In the first, there is blame. In the second, there is no blame, just acknowledgment and information. When complex emotions appear in your relationships, how are they managed? Give it some attention and notice your patterns. Are there situations it usually happens in? Does it come up more around certain sexual activities than others? What does it mean to experience disappointment (or any other heightened emotion)? Or to hear that your partner is disappointed? Once you spend some time unpacking why disappointment is a difficult emotion for you to handle, it becomes easier to create new patterns. Making room for disappointment means you're better able to manage yourself and your feelings when they matter. Developing greater emotional intelligence informs erotic intelligence, then potentially enables greater creative risk taking and more fun in the long term.

Suggestion: Identify exactly what you fear being disappointed about or how you might disappoint. Write down your expectations / concerns. Be specific. By avoiding disappointment or fear disappointing another, what are you missing out on? Weigh up the checks and balances. Is it a reasonable thing to be avoidant of or are the costs greater than the actual event itself? What's working well in your sex life? What areas are you confident about? If it's difficult to explore complex emotions with your partner, reach out to a therapist or coach who is skilled in these areas. Most people need support with emotional processing and developing emotional and erotic intelligence. Do not put it off for shame and embarrassment. It changes lives.

Pressure and Expectation
In addition to disappointment, people also experience pressure and expectation as passion killers. As we discovered in the early chapters of this book, because most of us didn't get a decent sex education, it's hard to know how diverse our palettes and interests are. While gender stereotypes die hard, even the most enlightened among us can still default to such narratives when attempting to make sense of complex sexual experiences. So alongside not wanting to disappoint, we can sometimes talk ourselves out of our desires because we preempt our partners' reactions based on the past, or based on ideas *we assume* about them because of fill-in-the-blank. For example, that one time you suggested watching porn and it was met with negativity? So you assumed that porn was forevermore off the table, when it could have simply been a case of bad timing, bad porn, bad manners, or bad luck. Unless we investigate and share what's really happening, we can find ourselves in a loop of misery forever based on misunderstanding. If we

never take the risk to speak about what we like and want, it never gets to be validated.

Conversely, we can enforce an erotic experience onto our partners by insisting, for example, that we are great at giving head because "none of my other partners ever complained." Such comments reduce the texture of subjective pleasure to assume that:

a. everyone loves receiving oral sex;
b. everyone loves the same kind of oral sex; and
c. all our previous partners were 100 percent honest about their erotic experiences with us and "there is absolutely no way s/he/ they would have lied or minimized their feelings or said nothing if they didn't *really* think I was fantastic at head."

Such stories from the past stop us from having meaningful and pleasure-centric sex in the present. When we expect our partners to react to sexual activities the way we would, or the way previous partners may (or may not) have, we can accidently create pressure around our connection which makes it hard to authentically connect.

Suggestion: Do you put pressure on your partner or yourself for sex to be or turn out a certain way? Do they put pressure on you? Talk about it. Use the methods from the previous chapter to take turns speaking and listening. Talk about the thing(s) that bug(s) you and try to get to the bottom of it. I assure you it will not fix itself, so do not be concerned if change takes effort. It does.

Are pressure and expectation things that apply in other areas of your life too? Do you tend to experience the world as a series of achievements—and this interferes with your capacity to enjoy yourself? Go back to your "why" about sex in chapter 6. Consider how these expectations help or hinder your whys, your conditions, and your erotic values (chapter 12).

Body Image

I'm too old and too fat for sex. Sex is for people who are more fill-in-the-blank. Oh dear! No matter how much we try, these ideas permeate our thoughts and, this far into reading this book, I *know* you now know why. People are going to find things about you sexy that you don't see, in the same way you're going to find sexiness in others that they don't see. Freckles, dimples, crooked teeth, saggy bellies, wonky eyes, hairy toes—you name it, someone's got it and someone else likes it. BUT . . . you are here for *you*, not for someone else's fetish or preferences. Here's the thing . . . you are not going to like every single thing about your body all the time, but it needn't ruin your entire approach to sex if you explore pleasure more broadly, as we've explored in this book. The whole *love yourself and say affirmations in the mirror* thing is great if it works for you—but it never worked for me. I felt fake and foolish saying shit I didn't believe. So, if you feel similarly, I see you. Don't get me wrong, I think body image matters a lot, but I think it matters in ways we haven't dedicated a whole lot of time to here. In the resources section of my website, you'll find authors whose works I admire and who specialize in things like aging, size, and disability. The truth is that your body image can really affect your desire and ability to enjoy yourself and you can learn to work with it rather than against it.

Suggestion: My good friend Elle Chase, author of *Curvy Girl Sex: 101 Body-Positive Positions to Empower Your Sex Life*,[4] suggests that instead of focusing on the things you hate, find things about your body that you like or feel neutral about. She suggests focusing on things like your hair color, eye shape, ankles, fingernails, and so on. Things and body parts that are not traditionally considered sexy, but still add to an overall aesthetic. Perhaps liking the way your body looks in certain positions is more helpful than loathing your body no matter what. If body image is holding you back from connecting with your body and pleasure, I urge you to reach out to Elle Chase for coaching and support.

Distraction

So many people who complain about the quality of their sex lives often remark that they do not know what they are thinking about or even doing *during* sex. It's like the lights are on but no one is home. And, we all do it. I do it. You do it. Everybody does it. It's completely normal and still very unpleasant and destructive when we are trying to build sexual connection to ourselves or others. Everything around us is designed to reduce our attention span to that of a gnat. Teaching yourself to stay present during sex is a practice, especially if you're new to it. For some people, a regular meditation practice helps with this. For others, it's yoga, Qi Gong, or some other physical activity that gives their mind a little respite too. Part of approaching it differently is first to recognize when it's happening and then address it in the moment, step-by-step. It's not a process of striving to make yourself perfect but a process of practicing keeping attention on what matters to you.

Suggestion: Look back at your sexual conditions (chapter 6), your values, and your sexual values (chapter 12). Review them to be sure they are still relevant. Add or remove any as necessary. These are effectively your accelerator as in the Dual Control Model introduced in chapter 5. Next, consider all the things that tend to distract you in the moment. These might be thoughts, feelings, or even activities.

In your notebook, respond to the following prompts:

- Things I **do** that distract me from my conditions and values are . . .
- Things I **think** that distract me from my conditions and values are . . .
- Things I **feel** (emotions *and* sensations) that distract me from my conditions and values are . . .
- When I am distracted from my conditions and values for too long, I feel . . .
- When I am connected to my conditions and values more often, I feel . . .

Make a commitment to focus more on what you want and less on what distracts you by working on ways to relax and destress in non-sexual contexts as much as sexual ones.

Trauma and Safety

Sexual trauma is rife. This is a social problem that affects the lives of individuals worldwide. Trauma happens in the form of sexual violence, but it also happens in the form of neglect, coercion, verbal and emotional abuse, and a lack of information about sex, pleasure, and health. Trauma is embedded in the way we are forced to disconnect from ourselves in order to survive. Trauma can manifest in many ways, including polarized thinking and a lack of ability to be present, feel feelings, and surrender to pleasure. As mentioned in the introduction to this book, I did not intend for it to be a trauma manual. The subject is so rich and complex I couldn't do it justice here. That said, many of the practices and approaches I offer are applicable to people living with the effects of sexual trauma too. If sexual trauma is impacting your capacity to enjoy your body and life, know that you are not alone and it's not your fault. Change is possible when you are ready.

Labels and Identities

Labels and identities help us find meaning in the world. Whether we are kinky, queer, gay, straight, or something else entirely, identity helps shape who we are and, perhaps to some extent, what we do. Sometimes though, our identities can begin to form a cage around us. Instead of giving us meaning, solidarity, and community, identity can stop us from experiencing pleasure for its own sake. For example, a gay man occasionally, or frequently, enjoying straight porn may begin to question his experience of pleasure because of its conflict with his identity. Straight men may be reluctant to enjoy anal sex because of the cultural association with homosexuality rather than receiving as an act of pleasure. Like many of the other examples in chapter 11, what brings us *pleasure* may sit in contrast with how we expect ourselves to be or behave. This tension is what sits at the heart of Morin's Erotic Equation: Attraction + Obstacles = Excitement (chapter 3). Be attentive to how tightly you hold your labels and the effect they have on your ability to open up to pleasure and ecstasy. Whether it's gender, orientation, practice, or some other label—they are there to work for you, not in spite of you.

Suggestion: Consider the labels you use to describe your gender, orientation, relationship style, relationship status, body, spirituality, diet, culture, nationality, and so on. Write them in your notebook and reflect on what these words imply about how you should behave sexually in contrast with how you feel, things you (might like to) do sexually or how you behave. For example, the identity of "mother," for many, brings up notions of chastity and virtue, even though, traditionally, the way one becomes a mother is primarily through sex itself. Of course, these days there are multiple ways to become a parent and even the identity of "parent" carries weight, but likely different in tone to the label "mother." For other people, the identity of "monogamous" can disrupt a couple's capacity to consider opening an otherwise loving relationship as a pathway through a stale sex life. While nonmonogamy is not for everyone, many more people are choosing consensual nonmonogamy as a way of invigorating a relationship that has lost its sexual sparkle. (My website lists resources for more information about opening up a relationship as a way of invigorating a tired sex life.) When you have explored your lists, consider how these may or may not be affecting your ability to show up in your body sexually and the degree to which these labels offer you meaning, support, and community or if you can expand them to also allow for robust eroticism, pleasure, and joy.

Perimenopause and Other Hormonal Malarkey

Are you in it? I am and it's awful, isn't it? As mentioned previously, I am not a medical expert, nor am I am menopause expert, but it's understood that while hormones can and do affect us in a variety of ways, it's not always a death sentence for your sex life. Heather Corinna, author of *What Fresh Hell Is This? Perimenopause, Menopause, Other Indignities, and You*[5] takes a deep dive into the effects of hormones on all aspects of our lives including sex. While discomfort and bodily changes as the result of hormones make things different and certainly difficult for some of us more than others, there is ample evidence that for those who want to resume fulfilling sex after an initial period of transition, it's infinitely doable.

Suggestion: Check the resources in Heather Corinna's book and head to my website for more information.

Desire Is Where You Find It

Learning to take care of your sex life is an ongoing relationship with life. Through these chapters we have taken the time to look at sex, emotions, pleasure, and what makes sex great for you today. And know that all this is subject to change as you change. As life changes. This is perfectly normal. There will be times your interest in sex waxes and wanes for no obvious reasons. The focus is always returning to your new tools and resources for finding the best way through. Even after twenty years of studying sex and discussing it with thousands of people, my relationship with it changes often. From now on, when you think about "normal sex"—please think about this. Recognize that change is the constant when it comes to sex, and with that we have the power to manage our sex lives and create the connections we most long for. When we can live with the ambiguity, when we can accept the uncertainty, when we can tolerate the insecurity sex brings up for us, we are in a better position to rise to the challenges it offers. When we can accept that the tension posed by sex for anything other than procreation is part of what makes it remarkable, we might be able to find what we are looking for and sustain it just a little bit longer. As I said before, and I'll say again, sex is not a problem to be solved but a quest to be seized. Undertake to do it deliberately and watch the sparks fly.

Notes

Introduction

1. Matthew Kelly, "You're your Dreams: The Answer to What Really Drives Employees," *Forbes*, August 21, 2019, https://www.forbes.com/sites/forbes coachescouncil/2019/08/21/in-your-dreams-the-answer-to-what-really-drives -employees/. *Good Morning America*, https://www.goodmorningamerica.com/ wellness/story/doctors-intimacy-anorexia-leading-sexless-marriages-65969306

2. Rebecca Jennings, "Dating Apps Are Everywhere: Relationship Apps Are for What Comes Next," *Vox*, September 11, 2019, https://www.vox.com/ the-goods/2019/9/11/20853452/couple-app-relationship-lasting.

Chapter 2

1. Pleasure Is the Measure https://fs.blog/knowledge-podcast/emily-nagoski/
2. Kate Bornstein, *My Gender Workbook: How to Become a Real Man, the Real You, or Something Else Entirely* (New York: Routledge, 1997).
3. Dawson, Samantha J. Dawson and Meredith L. Chivers. "Gender Differences and Similarities in Sexual Desire." *Current Sexual Health Reports* 6, no. 4 (2014): 211–19. https://doi.org/10.1007/s11930-014-0027-5.
4. Sarah H. Murray, Robin Milhausen, Cynthia Graham, Leon Kuczynski, "A Qualitative Exploration of Factors That Affect Sexual Desire among Men Aged 30 to 65 in Long-Term Relationships," *The Journal of Sex Research* 54, no. 3 (2016): 1–12.

5. Murray, Milhausen, Graham, and Kuczynski, "A Qualitative Exploration of Factors That Affect Sexual Desire among Men Aged 30 to 65 in Long-Term Relationships."

6. Dawson and Chivers, "Gender Differences and Similarities in Sexual Desire."

7. Dawson and Chivers, "Gender Differences and Similarities in Sexual Desire."

8. Katrien Wierchx, Els Elaut, Birgit Van hoorde, Gunter Heylens, Griet De Cuypere, Stan

M. Monstrey, Steven Weyers, Piet Hobeke, and Guy T'Sjoen, "Sexual Desire in Trans Persons: Associations with Sex Reassignment Treatment," *Journal of Sexual Medicine* 11, no. 1 (2014): 107–18. https://doi.org/10.1111/jsm.12365.

9. Lucie Fielding, *Trans Sex.* (New York: Routledge, 2021).

Chapter 3

1. Jack Morin, *The Erotic Mind: Unlocking the Inner Sources of Passion and Fulfillment* (New York: HarperCollins, 1995).

2. Lewis, C. S. *The Allegory of Love: A Study in Medieval Tradition.* (Oxford: Clarendon Press, 1936).

3. Simon May, *Love: A History*, Kindle edition (New Haven, CT: Yale University Press, 2011).

4. Stephanie Coontz, *Marriage, A History: How Love Conquered Marriage*, Google Books edition (New York: Penguin, 2006), 16.

Chapter 4

1. Peggy J. Kleinplatz and A. Dana Ménard, *Magnificent Sex: Lessons from Extraordinary Lovers* (London: Taylor & Francis, 2020).

2. Leonore Teifer. *Sex Is Not a Natural Act and Other Essays* (Boulder, CO: Westview Press, 2004).

3. William Masters and Virginia E. Johnson, *Human Sexual Reponse* (Boston: Little, Brown and Company, 1966).

4. Rosemary Basson, "Human Sex Response Cycles," *Journal of Sex and Marital Therapy* 27, no. 1 (2001): 33–43.

5. Helen Singer Kaplan, "Hypoactive Sexual Desire," *Journal of Sex and Marital Therapy* 3, no. 1 (1977): 3–9. https://doi.org/10.1080/00926237708405343.

Chapter 5

1. Katherine L. Goldey and Sari M. van Anders, "Sexual Arousal and Desire: Interrelations and Responses to Three Modalities of Sexual Stimuli," *Journal of Sexual Medicine* 9, no. 9 (2012): 2315–29.

2. Deanna Carpenter, Erick Janssen, Cynthia Graham, Harrie Vorst, and Jelte Wicherts, "Women's Scores on the Sexual Inhibition / Sexual Excitation Scales (SES/SIS): Gender Similarities and Differences," *The Journal of Sex Research* 41, no. 1 (2008): 36–48.

3. John Bancroft, "Sexual Desire and the Brain Revisited," *Sexual and Relationship Therapy* 25, no. 2 (2010): 166–71.

4. Bancroft, "Sexual Desire and the Brain Revisited."

5. Emily Nagoski, *Come As You Are: The Surprising New Science That Will Transform Your Sex Life* (New York: Simon & Schuster, 2015), 46.

6. James Pfaus, "Pathways of Sexual Desire," *Journal of Sexual Medicine* 6, no. 6 (2009): 1506–33.

7. To take an introductory assessment in determining your individual SES and SIS, the Kinsey Institute offers an online test as part of an ongoing study at https://iukinseyinstitute.co1.qualtrics.com/jfe/form/SV _9LBtS5dal6c37Rr?survey_id=9dff4e9a3dd78f2c4cfb.

8. Bancroft, "Sexual Desire and the Brain Revisited."

9. Samantha J. Dawson and Meredith L. Chivers, "Gender Specificity of Solitary and Dyadic Sexual Desire Among Gynephilic and Androphilic Women and Men," *The Journal of Sexual Medicine* 11, no. 4 (2014): 980–94.

10. Diana Fosha, Daniel J. Seigel, and Marion F. Solomon, eds., *The Healing Power of Emotion: Affective Neuroscience, Development, Clinical Practice* (New York: W. W. Norton & Company, 2009).

11. Fosha, Seigel, and Solomon, *The Healing Power of Emotion.*

12. Fosha, Seigel, and Solomon, *The Healing Power of Emotion.*

13. Pfaus, "Pathways of Sexual Desire."

14. Bessel van der Kolk. *The Body Keeps the Score: Mind, Brain, and Body in the Transformation of Trauma* (New York: Penguin, 2014).

15. Fosha, Seigel, and Solomon, *The Healing Power of Emotion.*

Chapter 6

1. Cindy Meston and David Buss, "Why Humans Have Sex," *Archives of Sexual Behavior* 36, no. 4 (2007): 477–507.

2. Marty Klein, *Sexual Intelligence: What We Really Want from Sex and How to Get It* (New York: HarperOne, 2012).

Chapter 7

1. Peggy J. Kleinplatz, A. Dana Ménard, Marie-Pierre Paquet, Nicolas Paradis, Meghan Campbell, Dino Zuccarino, and Lisa Mehak. "The Components of Optimal Sexuality: A Portait of Great Sex." *The Canadian Journal of Human Sexuality* 18, nos. 1–2 (2009): 1–13.

2. Diana Fosha, Daniel J. Seigel, and Marion F. Solomon, eds., *The Healing Power of Emotion: Affective Neuroscience, Development, Clinical Practice* (New York: W. W. Norton & Company, 2009), Chapter 1.

3. Peggy J. Kleinplatz and A. Dana Ménard, *Magnificent Sex: Lessons from Extraordinary Lovers* (London: Taylor & Francis, 2020).

4. Lorde, Audre. *Uses of the Erotic: The Erotic as Power* (Brooklyn, NY: Out & Out Books, 1978), 88.

Chapter 8

1. Lucie Fielding, *Trans Sex* (New York: Routledge, 2021).

2. Nicholas J. Fox. *The Body* (London: Polity Press, 2012); https://www.amazon.com/Body-Nicholas-J-Fox/dp/0745651240

3. Bessel van der Kolk. *The Body Keeps the Score: Mind, Brain, and Body in the Transformation of Trauma* (New York: Penguin, 2014).

4. Seigel, Daniel J, Diana Fosha, and Marion Solomon. *The Healing Power of Emotion: Affective Neuroscience, Development & Clinical Practice* (New York: W.W. Norton & Co., 2009).

5. Bessel A. van der Kolk, *The Body Keeps the Score: Brain, Mind, and Body in the Healing of Trauma* (New York: Penguin, 2014); Pat Ogden, Kekuni Minton, and Clare Pain, *Trauma and the Body: A Sensorimotor Approach to Psychotherapy* (New York: W. W. Norton & Company, 2006).

6. Barnaby Barrat, *The Emergence of Somatic Psychology and Bodymind Therapy* (New York: Palgrave Macmillan, 2010).

7. Ogden, Minton, and Pain, *Trauma and the Body*.

8. Gendlin, Eugene. *Focusing* (London: Everest House, 1978).

Chapter 9

1. Betty Martin and Robin Dalzen, *The Art of Receiving and Giving: The Wheel of Consent* (Eugene, OR: Luminare Press, 2021).

2. Matthew Hertenstein, Rachel Holmes, Margaret McCullough, and Dacher Keltner, "The Communication of Emotion via Touch," *Emotion* 9, no. 4 (2009): 566–73, https://doi.org/10.1037/a0016108.

Chapter 10

1. https://barbaracarrellas.com/why-tantra-now/
2. *The Crash Pad*. Directed by Pink White Productions. www.thecrashpad-series.com.
3. Esther Perel, *Mating in Captivity: In Search of Erotic Intelligence* (New York: HarperCollins, 2006).
4. Diana Fosha, Daniel J. Seigel, and Marion F. Solomon, eds., *The Healing Power of Emotion: Affective Neuroscience, Development, Clinical Practice* (New York: W. W. Norton & Company, 2009).
5. Staci Haines, *Healing Sex: A Mind-Body Approach to Healing Sexual Trauma* (San Francisco, CA: Cleis Press, 2007).

Chapter 11

1. David M. Ortmann and Richard A. Sprott, *Sexual Outsiders: Understanding BDSM Sexualities and Communities* (Lanham, MD: Rowman & Littlefield, 2013).
2. Michael J. Bader, *Arousal: The Secret Logic of Sexual Fantasies* (New York: St. Martin's Griffin, 2003).
3. Charmaine Borg and Peter J. de Jong, "Feelings of Disgust and Disgust-Induced Avoidance Weaken following Induced Sexual Arousal in Women," *PLoS ONE* 7, no. 9 (2012): https://doi.org/10.1371/journal.pone.0044111.
4. Justin Lehmiller, "Do Asexual People Maturbate and Have Sexual Fantasies?" *Sex & Psychology*, blog, posted January 31, 2015, https://www.lehmiller.com/blog/2015/1/31/do-asexual-people-masturbate-and-have-sexual-fantasies.
5. Justin Lehmiller, *Tell Me What You Want: The Science of Sexual Desire and How It Can Help You Improve Your Sex Life* (Boston, MA: Da Capo Lifelong Books, 2018).
6. Lehmiller, *Tell Me What You Want.*
7. Jack Morin, *The Erotic Mind: Unlocking the Inner Sources of Passion and Fulfillment* (New York: HarperCollins, 1995).
8. Morin, J. *The Erotic Mind: Unlocking the Inner Sources of Passion and Fulfillment* (New York: HarperCollins, 1995).

Chapter 12

1. The Gottman Institute www.gottman.com.

Chapter 13

1. Brené Brown, "Shame vs. Guilt," brenebrown.com, blog, posted January 14, 2013, Accessed August 13, 2021. https://brenebrown.com/blog/2013/01/14/shame-v-guilt/.

2. Joan Price, *The Ultimate Guide to Sex After 50: How to Maintain—or Regain—A Spicy, Satisfying Sex Life* (New York: Cleis Press, 2015).

3. JoEllen Notte, *The Monster Under the Bed: Sex, Depression, and the Conversations We Aren't Having* (Portland, OR: Thorntree Press, 2020).

4. Elle Chase, *Curvy Girl Sex: 101 Body-Positive Positions to Empower Your Sex Life* (Beverly, MA: Fair Winds Press, 2017).

5. Heather Corinna, *What Fresh Hell Is This? Perimenopause, Menopause, Other Indignities, And You* (New York: Hachette Books, 2021).

Bibliography

Bader, Michael J. *Arousal: The Secret Logic of Sexual Fantasies*. New York: St. Martin's Griffin, 2003.

Bancroft, John. *Human Sexuality and Its Problems*, third edition. Edinburgh: Churchill Livingstone, 2009.

————. "Sexual Desire and The Brain Revisited." *Sexual and Relationship Therapy* 25, no. 2 (2010): 166–71.

Barrat, Barnaby. *The Emergence of Somatic Psychology and Bodymind Therapy*. New York: Palgrave Macmillan, 2010.

Basson, Rosemary. "Human Sex-Response Cycles." *Journal of Sex and Marital Therapy* 27, no. 1 (2001): 33–43.

Borg Charmaine, and Peter J. de Jong. "Feelings of Disgust and Disgust-Induced Avoidance Weaken Following Induced Sexual Arousal in Women." *PLoS ONE* 7, no. 9 (2012): https://doi.org/10.1371/journal.pone.0044111.

Bornstein, Kate. *My Gender Workbook: How to Become a Real Man, a Real Woman, the Real You, or Something Else Entirely*. New York: Routledge, 1997.

Brown, Brené. "Shame vs. Guilt." brenebrown.com. Blog. Posted January 14, 2013. Accessed August 13, 2021. https://brenebrown.com/blog/2013/01/14/shame-v-guilt/.

Carpenter, Deanna, Erick Janssen, Cynthia Graham, Harrie Vorst, and Jelte Wicherts. "Women's Scores on the Sexual Inhibition /Sexual Excitation Scales (SES/SIS): Gender Similarities and Differences." *The Journal of Sex Research* 41, no. 1 (2008): 36–48.

Chase, Elle. *Curvy Girl Sex: 101 Body-Positive Positions to Empower Your Sex Life*. Beverly, MA: Fair Winds Press, 2017.

Coontz, Stephanie. *Marriage, A History: How Love Conquered Marriage*. New York: Penguin, Kindle edition, 2006.

Corinna, Heather. *What Fresh Hell Is This? Perimenopause, Menopause, Other Indignities, and You*. New York: Hachette Books, 2021.

Dawson, Samantha J., and Meredith L. Chivers. "Gender Differences and Similarities in Sexual Desire." *Current Sexual Health Reports* 6, no. 4 (2014): 211–19. https://doi.org/10.1007/s11930-014-0027-5.

———. "Gender Specificity of Solitary and Dyadic Sexual Desire among Gynephilic and Androphilic Women and Men." *The Journal of Sexual Medicine* 11, no. 4 (2014): 980–94.

Fielding, Lucie. *Trans Sex*. New York: Routledge, 2021.

Fosha, Diana, Daniel J. Seigel, and Marion F. Solomon, eds. *The Healing Power of Emotion: Affective Neuroscience, Development, Clinical Practice*. New York: W. W. Norton & Company, 2009.

Fox, Nicholas. J. *The Body*. London: Polity Press, 2012; https://www.wiley.com/en-us.

Goldey, Katherine L., and Sari M. van Anders. "Sexual Arousal and Desire: Interrelations and Responses to Three Modalities of Sexual Stimuli." *Journal of Sexual Medicine* 9, no. 9 (2012): 2315–29.

Haines, Staci. *Healing Sex: A Mind-Body Approach to Healing Sexual Trauma*. San Francisco, CA: Cleis Press, 2007.

Hertenstein, Matthew. J., Rachel Holmes, Margaret McCullough, and Dacher Keltner. "The Communication of Emotion via Touch." *Emotion* 9, no. 4 (2009): 566–73. https://doi.org/10.1037/a0016108.

Janssen, Erick, and John Bancroft. "The Dual Control Model: The Role of Sexual Inhibition and Excitation in Sexual Arousal and Behavior." In *The Psychophysiology of Sex*, edited by Erick Janssen, 197–222. Bloomington: Indiana University Press, 2007.

Jennings, Rebecca. "Dating Apps Are Everywhere: Relationship Apps Are for What Comes Next." *Vox*, September 11, 2019. https://www.vox.com/the-goods/2019/9/11/20853452/couple-app-relationship-lasting.

Kaplan, Helen Singer. "Hypoactive Sexual Desire." *Journal of Sex and Marital Therapy* 3, no. 1 (1977): 3–9. https://doi.org/10.1080/00926237708405343.

Kelly, Matthew. "You're your Dreams: The Answer to What Really Drives Employees." *Forbes*, August 21, 2019. https://www.forbes.com/sites/forbescoachescouncil/2019/08/21/in-your-dreams-the-answer-to-what-really-drives-employees/.

Klein, Marty. 2012. *Sexual Intelligence: What We Really Want from Sex and How to Get It.* New York: HarperOne, 2012.

Kleinplatz, Peggy J., and A. Dana Ménard. *Magnificent Sex: Lessons from Extraordinary Lovers.* London: Taylor & Francis, 2020.

Kleinplatz, Peggy J., A. Dana Ménard, Marie-Pierre Paquet, Nicolas Paradis, Meghan Campbell, Dino Zuccarino, and Lisa Mehak. "The Components of Optimal Sexuality: A Portait of Great Sex." *The Canadian Journal of Human Sexuality* 18, nos. 1–2 (2009): 1–13.

Lehmiller, Justin. "Do Asexual People Maturbate and Have Sexual Fantasies?" *Sex & Psychology.* Blog. Posted January 31, 2015. https://www.lehmiller.com/blog/2015/1/31/do-asexual-people-masturbate-and-have-sexual-fantasies.

————. *Tell Me What You Want: The Science of Sexual Desire and How It Can Help You Improve Your Sex Life.* Boston, Da Capo Lifelong Books: 2018.

Martin, Betty, and Robin Dalzen. *The Art of Receiving and Giving: The Wheel of Consent.* Eugene, OR: Luminare Press, 2021.

Masters, William, and Virginia E. Johnson. *Human Sexual Reponse.* Boston: Little, Brown and Company, 1966.

May, Simon. *Love: A History.* Kindle. New Haven, CT: Yale University Press, 2011.

Meston, Cindy, and David M. Buss. "Why Humans Have Sex." *Archives of Sexual Behavior* 36, no. 4 (2007): 477–507.

Morin, Jack. *The Erotic Mind: Unlocking the Inner Sources of Passion and Fulfillment.* New York: HarperCollins, 1995.

Murray, Sarah H., Robin Milhausen, Cynthia Graham, Leon Kuczynski. "A Qualitative Exploration of Factors That Affect Sexual Desire among Men Aged 30 to 65 in Long-Term Relationships." *The Journal of Sex Research* 54, no. 3 (2016): 1–12.

Nagoski, Emily. *Come As You Are: The Surprising New Science That Will Transform Your Sex Life.* New York: Simon & Schuster, 2015.

Notte, JoEllen. *The Monster Under the Bed: Sex, Depression, and the Conversations We Aren't Having.* Portland, OR: Thorntree Press, 2020.

Ogden, Pat, Kekuni Minton, and Clare Pain. *Trauma and The Body: A Sensorimotor Approach to Psychotherapy.* New York: W. W. Norton & Company, 2006.

Ortmann, David M., and Richard A. Sprott. *Sexual Outsiders: Understanding BDSM Sexualities and Communities.* Lanham, MD: Rowman & Littlefield, 2013.

Perel, Esther. *Mating In Captivity: In Search of Erotic Intelligence.* New York: HarperCollins, 2006.

Pfaus, James. "Pathways of Sexual Desire." *Journal of Sexual Medicine* 6, no. 6 (2009): 1506–33.

Price, Joan. *The Ultimate Guide to Sex After 50: How to Maintain—or Regain—a Spicy, Satisfying Sex Life*. New York: Cleis Press, 2015.

Teifer, Leonore. *Sex Is Not a Natural Act and Other Essays*. Boulder, CO: Westview Press. 2004.

Thompson, Evan. "ISCS 2016—Closing Keynote—Evan Thompson." *Mind & Life Institute*, YouTube video, 1:03:55, posted December 6, 2016. https://www.youtube.com/watch?v=Q17_A0CYa8s.

van der Kolk, Bessel A. *The Body Keeps the Score: Brain, Mind, and Body in the Healing of Trauma*. New York: Penguin, 2014.

Wierckx, Katrien, Els Elaut, Birgit Van hoorde, Gunter Heylens, Griet De Cuypere, Stan M. Monstrey, Steven Weyers, Piet Hobeke, and Guy T'Sjoen. "Sexual Desire in Trans Persons: Associations with Sex Reassignment Treatment." *Journal of Sexual Medicine* 11, no. 1 (2014): 107–18. https://doi.org/10.1111/jsm.12365.

Index

124–25; in cultures, 124;
embodiment of, 174; in human
sexuality, 14–16; judgment and,
185; list of, 187–89; mapping,
189–91, *190*; motivations and,
191–92; notebook with personal,
124, 187–89; of pleasure, 19–20;
in relationships, 197; in Three-
Minute Game, 143; Time for
Reflection of cultural, 124;
trust and personal, 227–28;
understanding, 187–89. *See also*
personal values
van der Kolk, Bessel A., 125
venn diagram, 195, *196*
visceral experiences, 36, 39, 173
vocabulary, of sex, 39
vulnerability, 129, 149, 192–93

wants: from arousal, 74; from brain,
82–84; through communications,
221; in erotic template, 44;
reasons for being unwanted, 214–
15; sex, 91; sex with different,
106–7; spontaneity of, 216;
unwanted erotic thoughts and,
171–74

well-being system, 82
wellness industries, 41–42
West, Mae, 119
Western culture: bias in, 7; certainty
in, 152; desire in, 15; erotic
massage in, 147–50; fantasies in,
177–79; romantic love in, 39; sex
education in, 41–42
What Fresh Hell Is This? (Corinna),
236
Wheel of Consent Model: accepting
in, 141; allowing in, 141, 160;
quadrants of, *139*, 139–41; risk-
taking in, 150; serving in, 141,
148; sexual values in, 187; taking
in, 140; touch in, *139*, 139–41,
149, 162
White, Barry, 135
willingness, 112–14, 163, 204, 215
women: desire of trans, 31; gender
stereotypes of, 121–23; men as
opposites to, 68–70; queerness
and, 56–58; romance arousing,
152. *See also* cis women

~

About the Author

Cyndi Darnell is a sex and relationships therapist, clinical sexologist, and leading authority on desire and libido. Originally from Melbourne Australia, she now maintains a global practice from New York City where she offers consultations and coaching worldwide helping people resolve erotic quandaries and transform fear into freedom.